Developing and Utilizing Digital Technology in Healthcare for Assessment and Monitoring

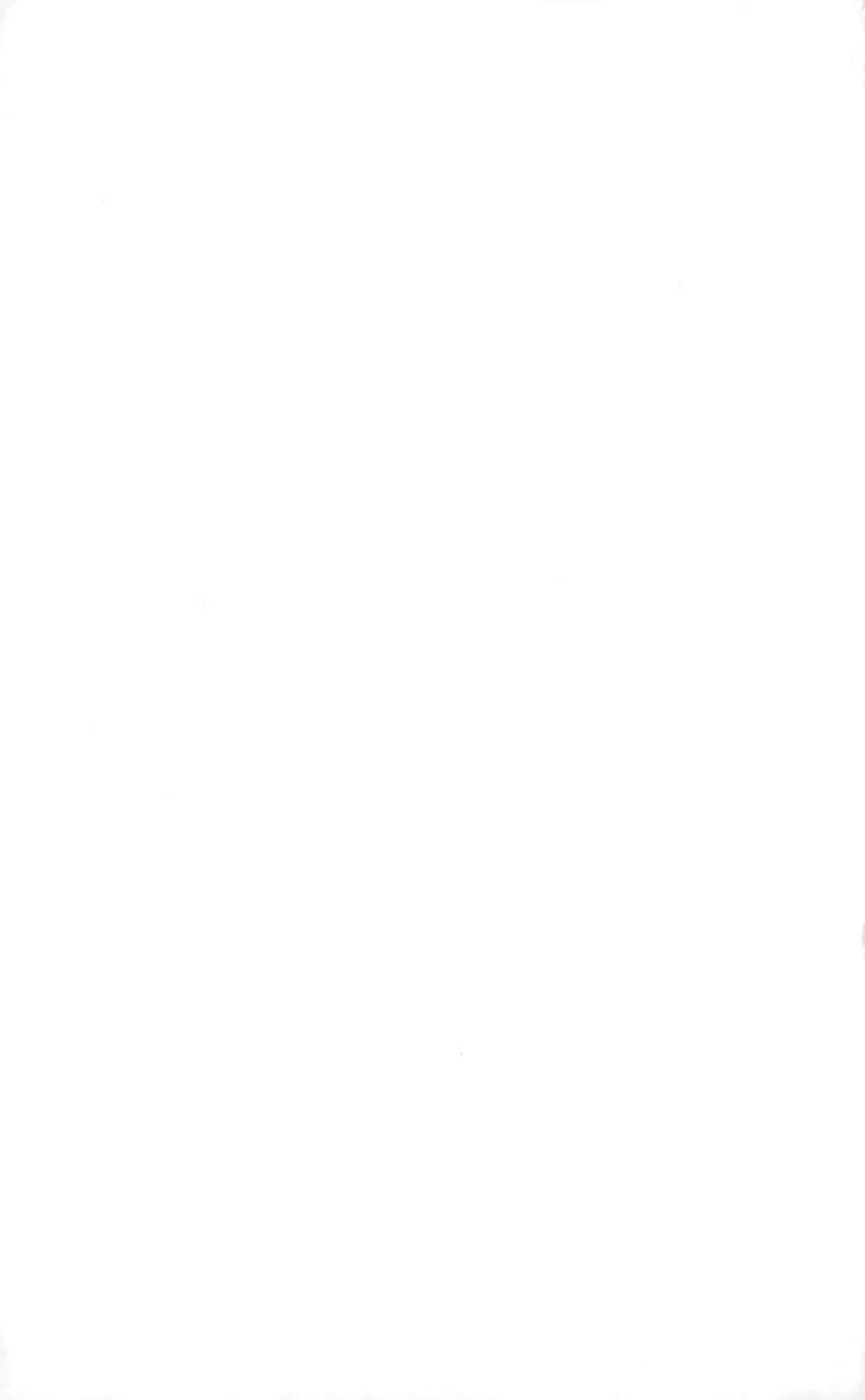

Andreas Charalambous

Editor

Developing and Utilizing Digital Technology in Healthcare for Assessment and Monitoring

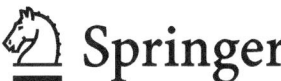 Springer

Editor
Andreas Charalambous
Nursing Department
Cyprus University of Technology
Limassol
Cyprus

ISBN 978-3-030-60696-1   ISBN 978-3-030-60697-8   (eBook)
https://doi.org/10.1007/978-3-030-60697-8

This Springer imprint is published by the registered company Springer Nature Switzerland AG
The registered company address is: Gewerbestrasse 11, 6330 Cham, Switzerland

Foreword

This very comprehensive book describes the potential of technology in improving healthcare and elegantly shows how these technologies can be utilized by many disciplines and professions in clinical practice.

In fact, the book is a multidisciplinary one, including nurses, academics, technicians, psychologists, etc. Actually, one of the first studies on the use of cellular phones to assist cancer patients at home was designed and conducted by a very active group of Scottish nurses, led by Nora Kearney, with the support of the company Vodafone, if I remember well. It was nearly 20 years ago and at the European School of Oncology we were very impressed by this idea, which then developed incredibly, in many other centres, into much more complex and advanced modalities.

I am sure many of you will remember the surprise generated by the appearance, in the corridors of the Memorial Sloan Kettering Cancer Center in New York, of the supercomputer Watson, developed by IBM to improve diagnosis of cancer patients.

As a surgeon, I will never forget the first time I saw a prostatectomy operation conducted by means of a Da Vinci robot: what a revolution! And what a deep change is currently happening in pathology, with the progressive introduction of digital pathology: have you ever thought of studying a slide by moving the mouse of your laptop rather than the knobs of your microscope? And to be able to send the images for a second opinion to your friend in Australia in just a few seconds?

The book is also very international. Authors come from the Netherlands, Switzerland, Cyprus, Canada, Ireland and Finland, reflecting the global nature of this area of research.

Only one warning comes to my mind in welcoming this excellent work: there is still a too big disproportion between our advances in technology and our competence in communication and relations with the patient. Medicine remains a very humanistic science, combining art and technology, passion and intelligence. In the foreseeable future no technology can yet replace the strength of a good, empathic

and personalized communication between the person who has lost the health and
the professionals of that health.

Alberto Costa
European School of Oncology
Milan, Italy

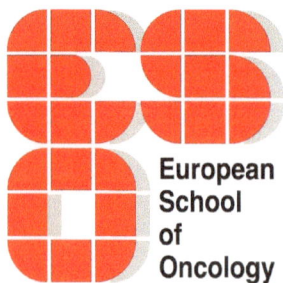

European
School
of
Oncology

Preface

The initial inspiration for this book came from a popular science fiction TV show and movie series *Star Trek* from the 1960s. Whilst there are numerous examples of gadgets that moved from science fiction to science fact, there is a device that stands out. This is the *Tricorder,* a multifunction handheld device used for sensor scanning, data analysis and recording data. Many of today's wearable sensors perform the same tasks and share the same features as the *Tricorder*.

What was seen 60 years ago as a science fiction has now become a reality in everyday living. Technology infiltrating in many fields of healthcare was seen as a natural development. The wider acceptance of these technological solutions has enabled their embracement within the healthcare context, as many devices such as the wearable sensors for example are both used by people as a daily lifestyle gadget and can also be used to extract health-related data for medical purposes. Artificial Intelligence, Virtual Reality, Augmented Reality, mobile applications, robots and telemedicine constitute only a fraction of the technologies that have been introduced in healthcare. Areas where these technological solutions have been utilized are also increasing rapidly. Symptom management, patient monitoring, surgical procedures and clinical decision-making support tools are now facilitated by technology.

The interest in the development and introduction of technological solutions in healthcare has never before received such an extensive attention. The shift of care provision to the outpatient context, health systems operating on limited resources and care becoming more complex are only some of the reasons that fuelled the research and development in this field. It is no longer considered a far reached luxury but on the contrary a necessity that is worth investing in.

This book brings together a wide range of authors from diverse disciplines and professions in an attempt to provide a comprehensive perspective to the topic at hand from development to utilization. As many of the technological solutions are addressed to patient users, the book provides an insight to personalizing this technological experience according to the user's needs and preferences. Similarly, as ethical concerns can be raised by the use of technology in healthcare, a chapter discusses this aspect in the context of social robots. Drawing on the expertise of field researchers the book provides their perspective in the utilization of technology as a means to manage symptoms and collect patient-reported outcomes. In the symptom management context, the book also explores the application of Virtual Reality, Augmented Reality and other digital interventions in clinical practice. Health games are accessible and enable reaching patients and clients without the restrictions of time and distance and are a valuable tool in healthcare. The book highlights recent research evidence on health games in healthcare, development and evaluation issues. The book also introduces IoT technologies that are utilized within healthcare in different environments: the in-hospital settings, the remote health services and the older adult care in home/nursing home settings. The challenges for implementing technological solutions in healthcare from an organizational perspective but also those challenges that emerge following the utilization of technology are presented to the reader.

This book echoes the many aspects of developing and utilizing technological solutions in healthcare. The book is therefore intended for researchers, developers (e.g., IT specialists), clinicians (nurses, physicians and other healthcare professionals) and different levels of students that are either working with patients across the care continuum or design and develop technological interventions for healthcare applications.

> We must continue to fight for funding for health technologies, so that they continue to do what they do best—save lives…
>   Albio Sires

Limassol, Cyprus   Andreas Charalambous

Contents

The Process of Developing Technological Solutions for Healthcare 1
Christos I. Ioannou and Marios N. Avraamides

Personalising the Technological Experience 19
Andreas Charalambous

Can a Robot Provide the Answer? Ethical Considerations
in Using Social Robots for Assessment and Monitoring in Healthcare . . . 29
Heike Felzmann

Development and Implementation of Patient-Reported
Outcome Measures in Cancer Care 45
André Manuel da Silva Lopes, Sara Colomer-Lahiguera,
and Manuela Eicher

Utilizing Technology to Manage Symptoms 55
Wendy H. Oldenmenger, Corina J. G. van den Hurk, and Doris Howell

Supporting Decision-Making Through Technology 73
Andreas Charalambous

Virtual Reality and Augmeneted Reality for Managing Symptoms 85
Andreas Charalambous and Androniki Ioannou

Using Internet of Things in Healthcare 105
Riitta Mieronkoski and Sanna Salanterä

The Use of Gaming in Healthcare 115
Anni Pakarinen and Sanna Salanterä

Implementation of Digital Health Interventions in Practice 127
Lisa McCann and Roma Maguire

Challenges and Future Directions: From Panacea to Realisation 143
Andreas Charalambous

The Process of Developing Technological Solutions for Healthcare

Christos I. Ioannou and Marios N. Avraamides

Introduction

Occupational or worked-related musculoskeletal disorders are widely common in the general population, affecting about 50% of all people. These disorders are characterized by pain symptoms deriving from musculoskeletal overuse, injuries or disorders of the muscles, nerves, tendons, joints, cartilage and spinal discs. Notably, in almost half of the affected individuals, this pain becomes chronic.

Occupations requiring extensive execution of repetitive motor activities under static postural positions and often under stressful conditions can induce occupational acute pain. Prolonged pain under the above conditions can neither be diagnosed specifically nor be associated with a strict pathology. However, its severity could keep affected individuals away from their professions [1].

One professional activity with probably the highest prevalence of musculoskeletal pain is playing a musical instrument with a 12-month prevalence up to 93% in professional musicians [2] and 67.8% in amateur musicians [3]. Pain symptoms of the musculoskeletal system generated while musicians are playing their musical instruments are known as "playing-related musculoskeletal pain" or just playing-related pain (PRP) [4, 5].

Performing a musical instrument which begins primarily before the age of 10 requires high temporo-spatial motor precision executed under sustained abnormal

C. I. Ioannou (✉)
Research Center on Interactive Media, Smart Systems and Emerging Technologies, Nicosia, Cyprus

M. N. Avraamides
Research Center on Interactive Media, Smart Systems and Emerging Technologies, Nicosia, Cyprus

Department of Psychology, University of Cyprus, Nicosia, Cyprus
e-mail: mariosav@ucy.ac.cy

© Springer Nature Switzerland AG 2020
A. Charalambous (ed.), *Developing and Utilizing Digital Technology in Healthcare for Assessment and Monitoring*,
https://doi.org/10.1007/978-3-030-60697-8_1

and un-ergonomically static postures mainly introduced just by holding the instrument. For instance, a violinist needs to hold both arms elevated with the left hand fully supinated. At the same time, the trapezius muscle generates force applied by the left chin to stabilize the instrument on the left shoulder. Under these conditions, a comprehensive control of the musculopostural parameters remains challenging and increases the risk of musculoskeletal pain deficits. At the same time, the daily practice (typically ranging from 3 to 5 h) required mainly by classical musicians induces muscular overloads and increases the risk of potential damage. Steinmetz et al. [6] reported that 93% of musicians diagnosed with playing-related musculoskeletal disorder showed dysfunction(s) of their postural stabilization system with females having higher vulnerability. In the same study, the authors supported that musicians who play more asymmetric movement patterns or instruments (e.g. violin) compared to non-asymmetric ones (e.g. playing the clarinet) can experience higher musculoskeletal pain problems [6, 7].

In addition to the level of motor precision required by instrument playing, professional musicians also expose themselves to an audience (e.g. concerts, competitions) which entails that their performance be not only flawless but also pleasant and entertaining. This often introduces (i.e. performance) anxiety and stress [4, 5, 8–10]. It is well known that performing under stressful conditions can introduce additional muscular tone that can accelerate fatigue, overuse and strain, and finally lead to the manifestation of PRP [11–14]. Furthermore, in chronic pain-affected musicians, the long period of disability and the difficulty to treat these conditions successfully often lead to the development of depression symptoms. Indeed, studies reveal an association between pain severity and depression among professional musicians [8] and between anxiety and pain among music students [15, 16].

Beyond abnormal postures and the muscular overexcitability due to the ergonomics of the different instruments and the overuse respectively, another factor that contributes to the musculoskeletal imbalances is the bad/incorrect practice routines (e.g. practicing with no breaks, "poor" physical conditions etc.) and the incorrect technical skill development. For instance, many musicians often exert additional and unnecessary muscular activity in order to press a string on a fingerboard or a key on a keyboard or by applying pressure with the thumb against the other fingers (i.e. tendency to hold the fingerboard of a string instrument with the left hand). Likewise, there is also a tendency for additional movements. Pianists, for example, often lift their shoulders during playing and violinists raise their upper right arm while using the bow. The tendency to produce unnecessary muscular activity and movement in addition to what is required contributes further to the development of musculoskeletal pain.

Overall, these physical and occupational playing-related conditions together with psychosocial pressures represent the main triggering factors for the manifestation of musculoskeletal pain symptoms in musicians. Therefore, improving postural positions to the maximum or eliminating unnecessary postural abnormalities and extensive or unnecessary muscular loads during instrument playing could contribute significantly to the prevention of PRP and increase performance to the maximum. However, playing a musical instrument is a complex activity that includes a number of unstandardized occupational parameters, making the generalization of preventive, diagnostic and treatment procedures inappropriate or only partly efficient.

Overview of the Current Obstacles Against PRP in Musicians

In a recent study, Ioannou et al. [15] found that about 60% of musicians who were diagnosed with chronic PRP continued to experience pain symptoms 2–3 years later even after receiving multiple treatments. This finding, together with the poor understanding of pain manifestation, indicates that there is a lack of well-preventive and reliable treatment approaches against PRP.

Although ongoing research aims to determine the pathophysiology of pain manifestation, a number of often-neglected occupational obstacles contribute significantly to the lack of well-established preventive, diagnostic and treatment procedures against PRP. For instance, in occupations that involve extensive engagement of the musculoskeletal system, such as in the case of instrumental musicians, the proper evaluation of the musculoskeletal mechanism should include assessment of both muscular and postural (motion) parameters. So far, the majority of the clinical evaluations of the musculoskeletal interactions consist of subjective opinions that are based on visual inspections. A more objective assessment of the potential interactions between muscular and postural mechanisms could provide a better understanding of the musculoskeletal mechanisms, especially during task execution. Furthermore, the majority of studies investigating training interventions of musculoskeletal parameters focus either on one of the two parameters or on specific body regions only [17–19]. Disregarding the full-body musculoskeletal mechanism is problematic as focusing onto one body region may unintentionally generate compensatory activity in other muscle groups. Therefore, the objective assessment of potential interactions between muscular and postural/movement parameters, which can be achieved via a simultaneous full-body recording of both, should be highly considered.

Another significant challenge is that, at least in non-severely affected musicians, pain symptoms develop primarily during playing the instrument. This is referred to as task specificity and it should be considered during the diagnosis and design of treatment procedures. The fact that a proper diagnosis should be conducted while musicians are playing their musical instruments was repetitively pointed out by specialized physicians [15]. However, this approach is not always feasible due to practical limitations (e.g. physical examination without the musical instrument) or lack of specialized physicians in the field of music [15]. However, as already mentioned, an objective evaluation of the musculoskeletal parameters (muscular asymmetry, overloads, etc.) during the execution of the instrument remains challenging, especially when deficits are subtle.

Furthermore, complexities against generalized PRP procedures derive also from the different biomechanics each instrument involves. For instance, wind instruments require activities and coordination primarily from the respiratory system, the mouth, the hands and the fingers. Furthermore, the way the sound is produced (e.g. airflow, pressure, tongue and lips positions/movements, facial muscles, etc.) differs significantly between trumpet, oboe and clarinet. In addition, the body posture also varies a lot. For instance, between a bassoon and a flute player, different postures, movements and groups of muscles are required. Similarly, differences exist across string instruments (violin vs. cello vs. contrabass) and across other instruments as well (e.g. piano vs. guitar vs. percussions etc.). These different demands provide an important challenge that makes imperative the development of more flexible and individualized preventive, diagnostic and treatment approaches against PRP symptoms in musicians.

Apart from the different structures and biomechanics required for each instrument, another important obstacle is the execution of the diverse music elements. Playing an instrument is a task which involves thousands of different movements, motor patters and combinations. Their operation depends on features related to dynamics (i.e. quite vs. loud sound), speed (slow vs. fast movements), different techniques concerning sound production (e.g. legato [tied together] vs. staccato [disconnected], simultaneous execution of several voices vs. monophonic melodies, etc.), sound duration (sustained notes vs. short notes), the number of repetitive patterns, etc. The execution of these different music elements, which also vary based on the different ergonomics of the instrument, requires variability of motion range and speed combined with activation of different muscular groups, muscular loads and endurances. Therefore, not only the execution of the instrument as an activity but also the task (musical content) should be taken into consideration during the development of musculoskeletal evaluations in musicians.

Beyond diagnostic assessments against PRP, healthy musicians or affected musicians undergoing a treatment retraining intervention also try to monitor their postural and muscular information while playing their instruments. Their aim is to minimize musculopostural imbalances and prevent the manifestation of PRP. To achieve this, healthy musicians often monitor themselves while playing in front of a mirror or by observing and imitating movements by other professionals or finally, by receiving (if available) feedback from a second observer (e.g. teacher). However, visual information reflected from a mirror or a second person is always limited and highly subjective. For instance, not all posture imbalances can be seen, mainly due to the asymmetric position the body already has when holding the instrument and occlusions that occur. Furthermore, while playing, musicians have to focus on musical-related elements (e.g. sound, pitch, notation, etc.) which may limit their visual or proprioceptive capacity to perceive information about their posture. Finally, no muscular activities (tensions, over-contractions) can be observed, neither from a second observer nor from a mirror. Instead, musicians must rely only on their proprioceptive awareness, which after a certain amount of time becomes weaker due to fatigue [18]. In light of these limitations, an objective and comprehensive tool allowing the self-observation of body posture and muscular activities during instrument playing could contribute significantly to PRP prevention and treatment procedures.

Apart from the above occupational and technical limitations, it has been reported that a comprehensive diagnosis and therapy against PRP should also include a psychological approach, especially in cases where pain symptoms become chronic [15]. Musicians, and especially those suffering from chronic pain conditions, could experience pain almost immediately after they start playing. The question which arises here is whether pain is a result of a particular pathology related to the musculoskeletal system or a cognitive (mis)perception deriving from malfunctioning neuroplasticity such as abnormalities in the primary somatosensory and motor cortex or grey matter reduction in the hippocampus and the amygdala [20–23]. One strategy against pain perception is cognitive distraction [24, 25]. Various distraction strategies (e.g. imagery, positive thinking, video games, etc.) against chronic pain have been widely used as potential psychological pain interventions, either on their own or as part of more elaborate cognitive behavioural therapies [26]. The challenge though with pain-affected musicians is to generate cognitive distraction while taking into consideration the various other challenges discussed earlier, i.e. training during the execution of the instrument, task specificity, the biomechanical demands of different instruments, etc. Even though the psychological extensions of pain in musicians is beyond the purpose of the current chapter, providing technological solutions which take into consideration all the above challenges would also encourage the development of more task-related psychological interventions against PRP.

Taking into account the limitations and challenges in the field of PRP in musicians, the aim is to develop advanced technological tools to provide dynamic assessments of the musculoskeletal mechanism while taking into consideration: (a) the simultaneous assessment of muscular and postural parameters aiming to provide understanding via objective data of potential interactions, (b) task specificity, meaning diagnostic assessments during the execution of the instrument, (c) diverse biomechanics required from the various instruments and musical elements, (d) real-time observation of the musculoskeletal parameters during playing the instrument, aiming to increase prevention and self-awareness against PRP, (e) multisensory feedback information offering the possibility to observe the musculoskeletal features from several viewing angles and (f) keeping musicians well motivated and engaged during preventive and/or treatment procedures. Considering these factors, which may depend on each other, in future procedures dealing with musculoskeletal assessments in healthy and PRP-affected musicians may lead to improved preventive, diagnostic and treatment protocols as well.

New Technologies for PRP

The optimal assessment procedure according to our approach is to observe on a display the body of the musician while playing the instrument, augmented with additional useful information. For instance, muscular activity could be visualized with heat maps at the various parts of the displayed body allowing the musician or a clinician to observe how muscular contractions change with the different movements of the body. Moreover, information concerning the postural behaviour (e.g. postural error deviations, axial rotations, etc.) and further muscular information concerning side-by-side muscular asymmetries, muscular overloads, etc. could also be projected on the display. Finally, the system could provide various viewing options such as observation from different angles, isolation of body regions, amount of diagnostic information displayed, etc., which could be selected according to the needs of the users.

The system sketched above could be implemented for two different ways, depending on the purpose. First, information from a session could be recorded and saved as an interactive video that could be used as a diagnostic tool by physicians. The video could provide different display options that a physician can select depending on what information is relevant to the diagnosis. The second way is to provide the information in real time. Such an implementation would be useful for healthy musicians (or affected musicians during treatment procedures) as it will help them to develop preventive strategies or follow treatment protocols. Again, the users can have the option to select the type and amount of information to be displayed.

To develop such an assessment tool that fulfils all requirements and overcomes the majority of the current diagnostic limitations in the field, we need to examine the effectiveness of existing tools and explore the possibility of adapting them to our specifications. In particular, existing (bio)feedback technologies related to electromyographic and postural/movement assessments should be thoroughly scrutinized. Also, since our approach entails visualizing and interacting with information on a digital display, existing virtual reality and augmented reality tools and relating technologies such as motion capture should also be explored.

The real-time observation of our own biological information (e.g. muscle tension, heart rate, skin conductance, respiration, etc.) translated into meaningful cues provided either visually, tactile or acoustically is known as biofeedback. Past studies have used biofeedback therapy primarily to restore motor deficits in upper and lower extremities mainly in stroke patients, as well as in traumatic brain injury, cerebral palsy and spinal cord injury. The benefits of biofeedback have been widely demonstrated in self-regulation procedures, during the development of preventive strategies (e.g. self-awareness, self-training, coping strategies), and during rehabilitation programmes that help patients to voluntarily gain control of various physiological functions [27–30]. In clinical research, the neuromuscular system has been widely studied with electromyography (EMG) in order to develop interventions that allow reducing muscle tension or improving muscle balance [31, 32]. Real-time biofeedback has also been used to improve postural stabilization (or balance training) in healthy young and adult populations as well as patients with Parkinson's disease, lower-limb surgery patients, after-stroke patients, patients with specific vestibular deficits and low back chronic pain patients [33–37]. Vuillerme et al. [38] suggested that the positive effects of the biofeedback postural stabilization training lie within the ability of the central nervous system to integrate biofeedback sensory information during training. In one study, Yasuda et al. [39] found that a balance training task was more effective when accompanied with haptic-based biofeedback. Interestingly, performance on a serial subtraction task carried out concurrently with the balance training task indicates no differences between the biofeedback group and a control, suggesting that biofeedback during motor training does not increase cognitive load substantially [39]. Finally, biofeedback has been shown to be effective against pain conditions, such as chronic headache, temporomandibular disorders, fibromyalgia and against psychological disorders (e.g. depression, cognitive coping) associated with chronic pain [28, 40–43].

Biofeedback has been also integrated in many cognitive behavioural therapies and was recognized as an effective part of rehabilitation primarily against chronic pain conditions. In some studies, it was reported that biofeedback treatment was even more successful than cognitive behavioural therapies in reducing pain severity and producing changes on affective, cognitive and behavioural variables over the long term [44]. A meta-analysis across 21 biofeedback studies (18 used EMG-based biofeedback) reported that biofeedback training/treatment (alone or coupled with other psychological or physiotherapeutic interventions) against chronic back pain could significantly improve one of the following variables: pain intensity, disability, depression, cognitive coping and reduction of muscle tension. Furthermore, the same study reported greater reductions in pain-related disability, and larger effects in depression reduction, with extended biofeedback treatments [43].

With respect to virtual reality (VR) tools, a few studies have already demonstrated their effectiveness as pain distractors against both experimental acute and chronic pain conditions (for a review see Malloy and Milling [45]). For instance, studies using virtual reality reported a decrease in pain intensity (and some of them improvement in anxiety) in patients suffering from burns [46–48], dental pain [49] and paediatric cancer [50]. In healthy individuals, virtual reality, in combination with opioid administration, was more effective than other control interventions, in reducing pain perception and pain-related brain activity against thermal pain stimulation [28]. In a more recent study, the performance of an isometric bicep curl training presented within a virtual reality environment reduced exercise-induced pain and increased time of exhaustion [51]. Overall, a number of studies have documented that VR could comprise a nonpharmacological form of analgesia, commonly referred to as "VR analgesia" (for a review see Mahrer and Gold [52]).

The real-time projection of visual feedback about movement on a virtual body has been so far rarely used in training protocols against pain, although it can provide valuable information for the immediate neuromuscular alterations related to postural and movement features [53]. In one of a few studies, Alemanno et al. [54] used audiovisual augmented feedback projected on a full-body animated character in an effort to reduce pain in low back chronic pain patients. Patients underwent a 6-week training aiming to regain a correct body image by observing the animated avatar presented in front of them. Results revealed significant pain reduction accompanied by improvements in quality of life, mood and functional abilities. A more recent study by Marshall et al. [55] examined whether visual augmented (bio)feedback combined with traditional lower extremity exercises can improve single-legged landing mechanics in female patients with medial knee displacement. Patients in a biofeedback and a control group were asked to perform the same training exercises. However, during training, patients in the biofeedback group observed on a monitor a real-time digital skeletal model of their body segments. In addition, colours on the model changed according to the movement in order to provide additional assistance. Results showed that, compared to the control group, the visual biofeedback group exhibited immediate (after one training session) and larger improvements in aberrant kinematics. Both studies [54, 55] suggest that virtual reality mirror visual feedback therapy is a promising training tool against chronic pain.

Overcoming the Challenges of Existing Treatments

Based on previous studies, several limitations and suggestions related to biofeedback visualization, training tasks, musculoskeletal data collection and engagement have to be carefully considered for the development of a new assessment tool.

First, so far, majority of EMG-biofeedback activities were displayed in a simple analogue or digital format (e.g. lines, icons or simple beeps, auditory signals, tactile stimulations, etc.) [29, 30]. As suggested by Huang et al. [29], during the design of dynamic feedback, visualizing trajectories towards the endpoint would be more beneficial than simple numerical EMG values. Therefore, our approach concerning the visualization of biofeedback data is focused on adopting smart interactive elements such as the mirror visualization of the movement on a digital avatar figure with heat maps representing muscular activity.

Second, in past studies, patients learned to self-regulate the activity of a specific muscle during static positions or during movements unrelated to the daily or pain-source activities [56–58]. These studies showed that static EMG-biofeedback therapies may thus produce only specific and limited effects on motor function recovery. Recent opinions on motor control support that improvement in functional activities would benefit from task-oriented biofeedback therapy and should be connected to a specific functional goal related to the specific action execution [29]. Task-specific movement components during biofeedback engage the interaction of the task-specific neuromuscular system within the relevant functional context [59]. This suggests that any (re)training through biofeedback needs to be conducted while musicians are playing their musical instruments. This will give the opportunity to musicians (healthy and affected) and physicians to develop dynamic observations and diagnoses, respectively, and further the knowledge of the musculoskeletal behaviour within the specific occupational context.

Third, in the very few EMG-biofeedback studies that have been conducted in musicians biofeedback was focused on specific body regions/muscles, without considering the overall full-body musculoskeletal mechanism [17, 60]. This has also been the case in studies on other populations using biofeedback on postural stabilization or posture. In these studies, assessments were conducted mainly by recording the centre of pressure or centre of mass [61], focusing mainly on pain intensity and range of motion [34]. However, none of the EMG postural biofeedback studies have examined muscular and postural/movement activity simultaneously. Especially in the field of occupational (task-specific) pain disorders, where pain manifestation and treatment depend on the characteristics of the work-related activity, data about musculopostural interactions could provide additional dynamic information. Based on the positive outcomes with respect to EMG and postural biofeedback training against pain symptoms, our suggestion is to combine these two elements to investigate the potential interrelations between them during action execution.

A final challenge in a successful biofeedback system is to provide as much relevant information as needed by the users and at the same time to keep them motivated and engaged during preventive or treatment procedures [29, 59, 62]. A recent study revealed that pain-affected musicians prefer to be actively involved in their treatment procedures as compared to passive pharmacological approaches such as consumption of pain killers [15]. Therefore, we believe that musculoskeletal (bio)feedback information visualized on a full-body virtual character would engage and motivate musicians and physicians to interact extensively with the system [54, 55].

Based on previous reports emphasizing the effectiveness of virtual reality, augmented reality, electromyographic and postural biofeedback training as individual tools against muscular and postural control and against pain symptoms, it seems that the integration of these technologies into a new tool is an optimal solution for providing preventive, diagnostic and treatment services against PRP in musicians. This approach can overcome the main challenges observed in treating not only PRP but also conditions in the entire spectrum of task-specific occupational musculoskeletal (pain) disorders.

Our Approach

Following the careful consideration of challenges and constraints stemming from (a) the nature of the specific medical field, (b) the needs of patients and physicians, and (c) the available related technologies, we have drafted a specific theoretical concept for a new tool. This tool is envisioned to serve two functions: (1) as a diagnostic tool to augment the procedures used by physicians, and (2) as a biofeedback tool to help healthy or affected musicians with prevention and treatment, respectively. For the implementation a concise design is recommended (see also Fig. 1) based on the following steps:

1. The integration of wireless EMG electrodes applied on the main body torso and limb muscles with wireless inertial measurement unit (IMU) sensors for motion capture attached to the respective body regions and joints, to simultaneously record muscular activities, posture and body movements. An easily used, adjustable and wearable suit allowing the quicker application of the EMG electrodes and IMU sensors could be considered.

2. The development of a virtual character that simulates the main physical characteristics of the user (e.g. height, weight, gender) and is animated in real time based on the user's movement. Additional visual (or auditory) information such

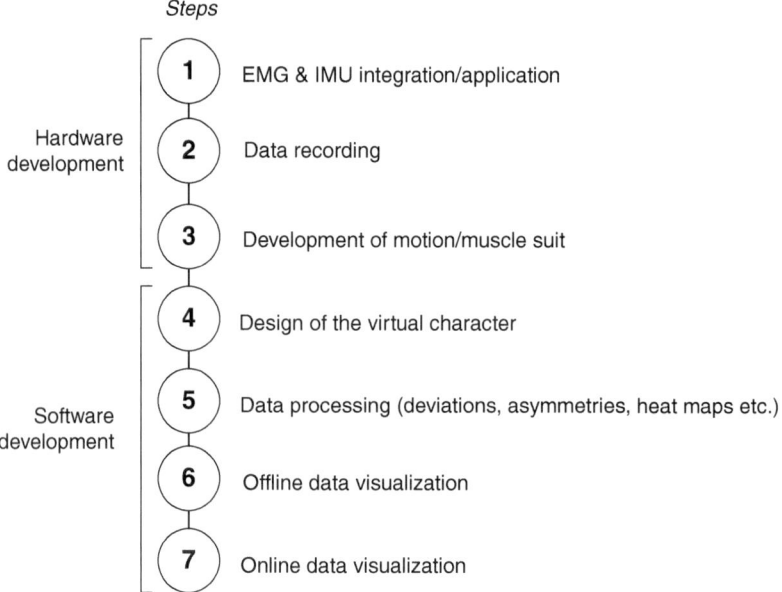

Fig. 1 Steps for developing a diagnostic biofeedback system for PRP in musicians

as visual trajectories, endpoints, equilibrium lines and muscular contractions projected will also be designed.

3. The design of a tool that will convert the musculoskeletal data into an offline diagnostic video that physicians can watch for diagnostic purposes. This will include (a) the character simulating the body movement of the musician, (b) the musculopostural diagnostic feedback parameters and (c) the audio produced by the instrument execution. Various options for customization according to the needs of the physicians will be implemented, e.g. selecting the observation angle, isolating specific body regions, presentation of averaged data based on timing information, etc.

4. The design of an additional tool that will provide biofeedback data in real time, to be used for preventive and treatment purposes. Through this tool, musicians will be able to observe their virtual selves in real time playing their instrument accompanied by feedback information about their musculoskeletal parameters. Again, various options for customization will be provided.

The proposed system allows observing accurate data about the muscular and postural parameters during the physical occupational activity. Diagnostic biofeedback information will be produced through mathematical and geometrical computations with respect to postural deviations, axial rotations, muscular over-contractions, side-by-side muscular asymmetries, etc. In the case of the diagnostic function, information will be converted and presented in an interactive video, available after a recorded session. This video will allow physicians to observe the performance and use the data to determine the sources of musculoskeletal pain symptoms, or other abnormalities while taking into consideration the abnormal positions necessary to hold each different instrument, and the postural and muscular alterations and inter-actions happening during the execution of the different instruments. Through the options provided, different metrics, such as muscle activity at different timestamps and viewing angles, could be chosen. The aim of the tool is to help physicians per-sonalize the diagnosis to each patient, problem and task.

The same musculoskeletal feedback parameters will be used for the biofeedback function, which will take place in real time. Users will observe on a display a virtual representation of their selves playing their musical instruments, augmented with real-time biofeedback data. This system can overcome the limitation of observing one's self in mirror by providing multiangle support and presenting proprioceptive information. The system will also be able to provide audio feedback to the user in the form of warning messages delivered through sound. This will alert the user for improper postures and other deviations when visual attention is occupied by other elements of task execution, such as reading the music notation. The system could provide a powerful tool for healthy musicians in order to develop self-awareness and knowledge on how their musculoskeletal system functions during instrument playing, allowing them to develop their own preventive strategies. For example, they could learn how to avoid unnatural or unnecessary movements that induce additional muscular loads, to correct improper technical routines, and to learn how the musculoskeletal system behaves when fatigue kicks in.

The biofeedback tool can be used by healthy musicians but also by PRP-affected musicians, as part of their treatment training programmes. It has been reported that, especially in musicians [63], observation of another person's movements activates neuronal activity in motor-related regions (known as "the mirror neuron system" [64, 65]). Therefore, our conjecture is that the observation of the virtual character (as in an actual mirror) imitating the movements of the user, together with the actual physical execution of the movement, would elicit higher neuronal activity and pro-duce greater impact and intensity during training. Finally, many chronic pain patients are characterized by a distortion of their body image and they often con-struct misleading perceptions about the physical state of their affected body region(s) [66–68]. We believe that observation of their (virtual) selves via such a biofeedback tool could also help them to recreate a proper body image and rebuild a more accu-rate perception of their actual physical state [54].

The suggested dual function system may overcome the majority of the chal-lenges musicians and physicians are currently facing while dealing with PRP (see Table 1). To summarize, postural and muscular parameters can be assessed together and in association with each other. The evaluation of musculoskeletal parameters for diagnostic purposes and for biofeedback through precise mathematical compu-tations will enable the provision of objective personal data. Assessment and diagno-sis can be conducted based on the execution of the actual task which triggers PRP, providing task specificity, while the biomechanics information characterizing the execution of different instruments and music elements is taken into consideration. Finally, the use of a VR-based display is associated with a number of important

Table 1 Current challenges solved by the development of the proposed diagnoses/biofeedback tool against playing-related pain in musicians

Purposes:	Prevention	Diagnoses	Treatment
Necessary for:	Healthy musicians	Physicians	PRP-affected musicians
Device functions:	Biofeedback	Diagnostic	Biofeedback
Current limitations concerning PRP in musicians			
1. Lack of correlation between postural and muscular properties	✓	✓	✓
2. Lack of subjectivity (need for objective reports)	✓	✓	✓
3. Lack of task specificity	N/A	✓	✓
4. Different instruments/demands	✓	✓	✓
5. Different motor patterns/activities (music elements)	✓	✓	✓
6. Observation of musculoskeletal activities in real time	✓	N/A	✓
7. Lack of multiangle observation	✓	✓	✓
8. Lack of proprioception information	✓	✓	✓
9. Ensuring engagement, interaction and motivation	✓	N/A	✓

PRP playing-related pain, *N/A* not applicable

benefits. For example: (a) all biofeedback information can be visualized without any interference from the different biomechanics of each instrumental and musical content, (b) the projected information can be focused on the problematic/affected body region(s) only or be isolated according to the information musicians (healthy or PRP-affected) wish to process simultaneously, and (c) the virtual character together with all the biofeedback information can be depicted and visualized from different view angles (e.g. anterior, posterior, lateral, etc.). On the one hand, the system can help patients develop their own self-awareness and pain management techniques during prevention and treatment interventions, respectively. Furthermore, such a system may keep musicians highly engaged and motivated during preventive or treatment procedures [69]. On the other hand, it may help physicians to arrange their diagnostic approach according to the features of the PRP and the individual characteristics of the patient.

Finally, a VR-based biofeedback tool such as the one described here could serve as a useful apparatus for researchers investigating occupational task-specific musculoskeletal pain disorders, especially in occupations requiring intensive repetitive motor tasks such as dance, sport, etc. Accessing multiple measurements during the execution of a task enhances ecological validity and may allow for better understanding the aetiology and manifestation (pathophysiology, biomechanics, etc.) of occupational musculoskeletal pain disorders. Moreover, with such a system, scientists can explore the musculopostural behaviour under the influence of different endogenous (e.g. psychosocial pressure, stress, anxiety, etc.) and exogenous (e.g. temperature, space, etc.) variables and develop personalized diagnostic and treatment protocols.

Conclusions

The estimated annual cost of work-related musculoskeletal disorders in EU is estimated at €476 billion per year, which is equivalent to the 3.3% of the GDP [70]. At the same time, pharmaceutical companies sound a note of warning about the crisis of drug abuse or misuse against chronic pain [71]. There is therefore great necessity for developing effective and flexible nonpharmacological treatments against pain disorders. Ideally, these treatments should adapt to the phenomenology and the needs of each individual patient in order to increase their effectiveness against worked-related musculoskeletal disorders. Here, we have described the concept for a technology-based tool that can help diagnose and treat occupational pain in musicians but can be also adapted for other professional groups. This tool can help physicians carry out data-informed individualized diagnoses and musicians to adopt preventive and treatment protocols. The next step to implementing the concept is to develop a prototype system. Then, rigorous laboratory testing is needed to evaluate the effectiveness of the system in achieving its intended purpose. The final aim is to bring to market a product that can really make a different in the field and a cost that would be attractive for consumer use.

References

1. Stock S, Nicolakakis N, Raïq H, Messing K, Lippel K, Turcot A. Underreporting work absences for nontraumatic work-related musculoskeletal disorders to workers' compensation: results of a 2007–2008 survey of the Québec Working Population. Am J Public Health. 2014;104:e94. https://doi.org/10.2105/ajph.2013.301562.
2. Kok LM, Haitjema S, Groenewegen KA, Rietveld ABM. The influence of a sudden increase in playing time on playing-related musculoskeletal complaints in high-level amateur musicians in a longitudinal cohort study. PLoS One. 2016;11:e0163472. https://doi.org/10.1371/journal.pone.0163472.
3. Kok LM, Groenewegen KA, Huisstede BMA, Nelissen RGHH, Rietveld ABM, Haitjema S. The high prevalence of playing-related musculoskeletal disorders (PRMDs) and its associated factors in amateur musicians playing in student orchestras: a cross-sectional study. PLoS One. 2018;13(2):e0191772. https://doi.org/10.1371/journal.pone.0191772.
4. Steinmetz A, Scheffer I, Esmer E, Delank KS, Peroz I. Frequency, severity and predictors of playing-related musculoskeletal pain in professional orchestral musicians in Germany. Clin Rheumatol. 2014;34:965–73. https://doi.org/10.1007/s10067-013-2470-5.
5. Ioannou C, Altenmüller E. Approaches to and treatment strategies for playing-related pain problems among Czech instrumental music students: an epidemiological study. Med Probl Perform Art. 2015;30:135–42. https://doi.org/10.21091/mppa.2015.3027.

6. Steinmetz A, Seidel W, Muche B. Impairment of postural stabilization systems in musicians with playing-related musculoskeletal disorders. J Manip Physiol Ther. 2010;33:603–11. https://doi.org/10.1016/j.jmpt.2010.08.006.

7. O'Shea C, Bettany-Saltikov JA, Warren JG. Effect of same-sided and cross-body load carriage on 3D back shape in young adults. Stud Health Technol Inform. 2006;123:159–63.

8. Kenny D, Ackermann B. Performance-related musculoskeletal pain, depression and music performance anxiety in professional orchestral musicians: a population study. Psychol Music. 2013;43:43–60. https://doi.org/10.1177/0305735613493953.

9. Spahn C. Treatment and prevention of music performance anxiety. Prog Brain Res. 2015;217:129–40. https://doi.org/10.1016/bs.pbr.2014.11.024.

10. Voerman JS, Klerk CD, Heyden KMV, Passchier J, Idema W, Timman R, et al. Pain is associated with poorer grades, reduced emotional well-being, and attention problems in adolescents. Clin J Pain. 2017;33:44–50. https://doi.org/10.1097/ajp.0000000000000367.

11. Ehrlenspiel F, Wei K, Sternad D. Open-loop, closed-loop and compensatory control: performance improvement under pressure in a rhythmic task. Exp Brain Res. 2010;201:729–41. https://doi.org/10.1007/s00221-009-2087-8.

12. Ioannou CI, Furuya S, Altenmüller E. The impact of stress on motor performance in skilled musicians suffering from focal dystonia: physiological and psychological characteristics. Neuropsychologia. 2016;85:226–36. https://doi.org/10.1016/j.neuropsychologia.2016.03.029.

13. Yoshie M, Kudo K, Ohtsuki T. Effects of psychological stress on state anxiety, electromyographic activity, and arpeggio performance in pianists. Med Probl Perform Art. 2008;23(3):120–32.

14. Yoshie M, Kudo K, Murakoshi T, Ohtsuki T. Music performance anxiety in skilled pianists: effects of social-evaluative performance situation on subjective, autonomic, and electromyographic reactions. Exp Brain Res. 2009;199:117–26. https://doi.org/10.1007/s00221-009-1979-y.

15. Ioannou C, Hafer J, Lee A, Altenmueller E. Epidemiology, treatment efficacy, and anxiety aspects of music students affected by playing-related pain: a retrospective evaluation with follow-up. Med Probl Perform Art. 2018;33:26–38. https://doi.org/10.21091/mppa.2018.1006.

16. Wristen BW, Fountain SE. Relationships between depression, anxiety, and pain in a group of university music students. Med Probl Perform Art. 2013;28(3):152–8.

17. Fjellman-Wiklund A, Grip H, Karlsson JS, Sundelin G. EMG trapezius muscle activity pattern in string players. Int J Ind Ergon. 2004;33:347–56. https://doi.org/10.1016/j.ergon.2003.10.007.

18. Neblett R, Mayer TG, Brede E, Gatchel RJ. Correcting abnormal flexion-relaxation in chronic lumbar pain: responsiveness to a new biofeedback training protocol. Clin J. 2010;26(5):403–9. https://doi.org/10.1097/AJP.0b013e3181d2bd8c.

19. Nord S, Ettare D, Drew D, Hodge S. Muscle learning therapy--efficacy of a biofeedback based protocol in treating work-related upper extremity disorders. Occup Rehabil. 2001;11(1):23–31. https://doi.org/10.1023/a:1016600107571.

20. Mutso AA, Radzicki D, Baliki MN, Huang L, Banisadr G, Centeno MV, et al. Abnormalities in hippocampal functioning with persistent pain. J Neurosci. 2012;32:5747–56. https://doi.org/10.1523/jneurosci.0587-12.2012.

21. Schmidt-Wilcke T, Gänßbauer S, Neuner T, Bogdahn U, May A. Subtle grey matter changes between migraine patients and healthy controls. Cephalalgia. 2008;28:1–4. https://doi.org/10.1111/j.1468-2982.2007.01428.x.

22. Thompson JM, Neugebauer V. Cortico-limbic pain mechanisms. Neurosci Lett. 2019;702:15–23. https://doi.org/10.1016/j.neulet.2018.11.037.

23. Yang S, Chang MC. Chronic pain: structural and functional changes in brain structures and associated negative affective states. Int J Mol Sci. 2019;20(13):3130.

24. McCaul KD, Malott JM. Distraction and coping with pain. Psychol Bull. 1984;95(3):516–33. https://doi.org/10.1037//0033-2909.95.3.516.

25. Wickens CD. Multiple resources and mental workload. Hum Factors. 2008;50:449–55. https://doi.org/10.1111/j.1468-2982.2007.01428.x.

26. Subnis UB, Starkweather A, Menzies V. A current review of distraction-based interventions for chronic pain management. Eur J Integr Med. 2016;8:715–22. https://doi.org/10.1016/j.eujim.2016.08.162.
27. Dupee M, Forneris T, Werthner P. Perceived outcomes of a biofeedback and neurofeedback training intervention for optimal performance: learning to enhance self-awareness and self-regulation with Olympic athletes. Sport Psychol. 2016;30:339–49. https://doi.org/10.1123/tsp.2016-0028.
28. Hoffman BM, Papas RK, Chatkoff DK, Kerns RD. Meta-analysis of psychological interventions for chronic low back pain. Health Psychol. 2007;26:1–9. https://doi.org/10.1037/0278-6133.26.1.1.
29. Huang H, Wolf SL, He J. Recent developments in biofeedback for neuromotor rehabilitation. Rehabil J Neuroeng Rehabil. 2006;3:11. https://doi.org/10.1186/1743-0003-3-11.
30. Pagé I, Marchand A-A, Nougarou F, Oshaughnessy J, Descarreaux M. Neuromechanical responses after biofeedback training in participants with chronic low back pain: an experimental cohort study. J Manip Physiol Ther. 2015;38:449–57. https://doi.org/10.1016/j.jmpt.2015.08.005.
31. Jung S, Lee K, Kim M, Song C. Audiovisual biofeedback-based trunk stabilization training using a pressure biofeedback system in stroke patients: a randomized, single-blinded study. Stroke Res Treat. 2017;2017:1–11. https://doi.org/10.1155/2017/6190593.
32. Neblett R. Surface electromyographic (SEMG) biofeedback for chronic low back pain. Healthcare. 2016;4:27. https://doi.org/10.3390/healthcare4020027.
33. Dozza M, Horak FB, Chiari L. Auditory biofeedback substitutes for loss of sensory information in maintaining stance. Exp Brain Res. 2007;178(1):37–48. https://doi.org/10.1007/s00221-006-0709-y.
34. Magnusson ML, Chow DH, Diamandopoulos Z, Pope MH. Motor control learning in chronic low back pain. Spine (Phila Pa 1976). 2008;33(16):E532–8. https://doi.org/10.1097/BRS.0b013e31817dfd9a.
35. Zijlstra A, Mancini M, Chiari L, Zijlstra W. Biofeedback for training balance and mobility tasks in older populations: a systematic review. J Neuroeng Rehabil. 2010;7:58. https://doi.org/10.1186/1743-0003-7-58.
36. Vuillerme N, Chenu O, Demongeot J, Payan Y. Controlling posture using a plantar pressure-based, tongue-placed tactile biofeedback system. Exp Brain Res. 2006;179:409–14. https://doi.org/10.1007/s00221-006-0800-4.
37. Vuillerme N, Chenu O, Pinsault N, Fleury A, Demongeot J, Payan Y. Can a plantar pressure-based tongue-placed electrotactile biofeedback improve postural control under altered vestibular and neck proprioceptive conditions? Neuroscience. 2008;155(1):291–6. https://doi.org/10.1016/j.neuroscience.2008.05.018.
38. Vuillerme N, Chenu O, Demongeot J, Payan Y. Controlling posture using a plantar pressure-based, tongue-placed tactile biofeedback system. Exp Brain Res. 2007;179(3):409–14. https://doi.org/10.1007/s00221-006-0800-4.
39. Yasuda K, Saichi K, Iwata H. Haptic-based perception-empathy biofeedback enhances postural motor learning during high-cognitive load task in healthy older adults. Front Med. 2018;5:149. https://doi.org/10.3389/fmed.2018.00149.
40. Glombiewski JA, Bernardy K, Häuser W. Efficacy of EMG- and EEG-biofeedback in fibromyalgia syndrome: a meta-analysis and a systematic review of randomized controlled trials. Evid Based Complement Alternat Med. 2013;2013:962741. https://doi.org/10.1155/2013/962741.
41. Moore A, Mannion J, Moran RW. The efficacy of surface electromyographic biofeedback assisted stretching for the treatment of chronic low back pain: a case-series. J Bodyw Mov Ther. 2015;19(1):8–16. https://doi.org/10.1016/j.jbmt.2013.12.008.
42. Nestoriuc Y, Rief W, Martin A. Meta-analysis of biofeedback for tension-type headache: efficacy, specificity, and treatment moderators. J Consult Clin Psychol. 2008;76(3):379–96. https://doi.org/10.1037/0022-006X.76.3.379.

43. Sielski R, Rief W, Glombiewski JA. Efficacy of biofeedback in chronic back pain: a meta-analysis. Int J Behav Med. 2017;24(1):25–41. https://doi.org/10.1007/s12529-016-9572-9.
44. Flor H, Birbaumer N. Comparison of the efficacy of electromyographic biofeedback, cognitive-behavioral therapy, and conservative medical interventions in the treatment of chronic musculoskeletal pain. J Consult Clin Psychol. 1993;61(4):653–8.
45. Malloy KM, Milling LS. The effectiveness of virtual reality distraction for pain reduction: a systematic review. Clin Psychol Rev. 2010;30(8):1011–8. https://doi.org/10.1016/j.cpr.2010.07.001.
46. Jeffs D, Dorman D, Brown S, Files A, Graves T, Kirk E, et al. Effect of virtual reality on adolescent pain during burn wound care. J Burn Care Res. 2014;35(5):395–408. https://doi.org/10.1097/BCR.0000000000000019.
47. Maani CV, Hoffman HG, Morrow M, Maiers A, Gaylord K, Mcghee LL, et al. Virtual reality pain control during burn wound debridement of combat-related burn injuries using robot-like arm mounted VR goggles. J Trauma. 2011;71(1 Suppl):S125–30. https://doi.org/10.1097/ta.0b013e31822192e2.
48. Das DA, Grimmer KA, Sparnon AL, McRae SE, Thomas BH. The efficacy of playing a virtual reality game in modulating pain for children with acute burn injuries: a randomized controlled trial [ISRCTN87413556]. BMC Pediatr. 2005;5(1):1. https://doi.org/10.1186/1471-2431-5-1.
49. Wiederhold BK, Gao K, Sulea C, Wiederhold MD. Virtual reality as a distraction technique in chronic pain patients. Cyberpsychol Behav Soc Netw. 2014;17(6):346–52. https://doi.org/10.1089/cyber.2014.0207.
50. Gershon J, Zimand E, Pickering M, Rothbaum BO, Hodges L. A pilot and feasibility study of virtual reality as a distraction for children with cancer. J Am Acad Child Adolesc Psychiatry. 2004;43(10):1243–9. https://doi.org/10.1097/01.chi.0000135621.23145.05.
51. Matsangidou N, Ang CS, Mauger AR, Intarasirisawat J, Otkhmezuri B, Avraamides NA. Is your virtual self as sensational as your real? Virtual reality: the effect of body consciousness on the experience of exercise sensations. Psychol Sport Exerc. 2019;41:218–24. https://doi.org/10.1016/j.psychsport.2018.07.004.
52. Mahrer NE, Gold JI. The use of virtual reality for pain control: a review. Curr Pain Headache Rep. 2009;13(2):100–9. https://doi.org/10.1007/s11916-009-0019-8.
53. Winstein CJ. Knowledge of results and motor learning: implications for physical therapy. Phys Ther. 1991;71(2):140–9. https://doi.org/10.1093/ptj/71.2.140.
54. Alemanno F, Houdayer E, Emedoli D, Locatelli M, Mortini P, Mandelli C, Raggi A, Iannaccone S. Efficacy of virtual reality to reduce chronic low back pain: proof-of-concept of a non-pharmacological approach on pain, quality of life, neuropsychological and functional outcome. PLoS One. 2019;14(5):e0216858.
55. Marshall AN, Hertel J, Hart JM, Russell S, Saliba SA. Visual biofeedback and changes in lower extremity kinematics in individuals with medial knee displacement. J Athl Train. 2020;55(3):255–64. https://doi.org/10.4085/1062-6050-383-18.
56. Bradley L, Hart BB, Mandana S, Flowers K, Riches M, Sanderson P. Electromyographic biofeedback for gait training after stroke. Clin Rehabil. 1998;12:11–22. https://doi.org/10.1191/026921598677671932.
57. Moreland JD, Thomson MA, Fuoco AR. Electromyographic biofeedback to improve lower extremity function after stroke: a meta-analysis. Arch Phys Med Rehabil. 1998;79:134–40. https://doi.org/10.1016/s0003-9993(98)90289-1.
58. Wolf SL, Catlin PA, Blanton S, Edelman J, Lehrer N, Schroeder D. Overcoming limitations in elbow movement in the presence of antagonist hyperactivity. Phys Ther. 1994;74:826–35. https://doi.org/10.1093/ptj/74.9.826.
59. Schmidt RA, Wrisberg CA. Motor learning and performance. 2nd ed. Champaign, IL: Human Kinetics; 2000. p. xii. 339.
60. Zinn ML, Zinn MA. Psychophysiology for performing artists. In: Schwartz MS, Andrasik F, editors. Biofeedback: a practitioners guide. 3rd ed. New York, NY: Guilford; 2003.

61. Keshner EA, Kenyon RV. The influence of an immersive virtual environment on the segmental organization of postural stabilizing responses. J Vestib Res. 2000;10(4-5):207–19. PMID: 11354434.
62. Weiss PL, Naveh Y, Katz N. Design and testing of a virtual environment to train stroke patients with unilateral spatial neglect to cross a street safely. Occup Ther Int. 2003;10(1):39–55. https://doi.org/10.1002/oti.176.
63. Haslinger B, Erhard P, Altenmüller E, Schroeder U, Boecker H, Ceballos-Baumann AO. Transmodal sensorimotor networks during action observation in professional pianists. J Cogn Neurosci. 2005;17(2):282–93. https://doi.org/10.1162/0898929053124893.
64. Rizzolatti G, Craighero L. The mirror-neuron system. Annu Rev Neurosci. 2004;27:169–92. https://doi.org/10.1146/annurev.neuro.27.070203.144230.
65. Rizzolatti G, Fadiga L, Fogassi L, Gallese V. Premotor cortex and the recognition of motor actions. Brain Res Cogn Brain Res. 1996;3(2):131–41. https://doi.org/10.1016/0926-6410(95)00038-0.
66. Förderreuther S, Sailer U, Straube A. Impaired self-perception of the hand in complex regional pain syndrome (CRPS). Pain. 2004;110:756–61. https://doi.org/10.1016/j.pain.2004.05.019.
67. Lewis JS, Kersten P, McCabe CS, McPherson KM, Blake DR. Body perception disturbance: a contribution to pain in complex regional pain syndrome (CRPS). Pain. 2007;133:111–9. https://doi.org/10.1016/j.pain.2007.03.013.
68. Moseley GL. I can't find it! Distorted body image and tactile dysfunction in patients with chronic back pain. Pain. 2008;140:239–43. https://doi.org/10.1016/j.pain.2008.08.001.
69. Sato K, Fukumori S, Matsusaki T, Maruo T, Ishikawa S, Nishie H, et al. Nonimmersive virtual reality mirror visual feedback therapy and its application for the treatment of complex regional pain syndrome: an open-label pilot study. Pain Med. 2010;11(4):622–9. https://doi.org/10.1111/j.1526-4637.2010.00819.x.
70. European Agency for Safety and Health at Work. An international comparison of the cost of work-related accidents and illnesses. https://osha.europa.eu/en/publications/international-comparison-cost-work-related-accidents-and-illnesses.
71. Cohen JP, Mendoza M, Roland C. Challenges involved in the development and delivery of abuse-deterrent formulations of opioid analgesics. Clin Ther. 2018;40:334–44. https://doi.org/10.1016/j.clinthera.2018.01.003.

Personalising the Technological Experience

Andreas Charalambous

Introduction

Technology is becoming the driving force that is changing the world at warp speed and nowhere is this more evident than in healthcare settings. While myriad forces are changing the face of contemporary healthcare, one could argue that nothing will change the way healthcare is practiced more than current advances in technology. Never has before the motto "*The future is now*" become so true in the everyday living of those at the recipient end of the healthcare but also at the delivering end of those providing the care. It is now recognised by many that technology has been instrumental in changing how healthcare works. Technology despite its rapid integration in healthcare still remains a tool of interaction between the provided and the user, and one that is designed to fulfil a user's needs. Therefore the management of long-term (and to some extent acute) conditions needs to be patient-centred, personalised, supporting patients in their homes (or/and other settings) and enabled by digital health, data analytics, behavioural science and connected medical devices.

Conceptualisation

Whilst in the literature there are many technological interventions that claim to have a personalised approach, a closer look reveals however a different story, making this a questionable claim. This is mainly due to the fact that these technologies describe

A. Charalambous (✉)
Nursing Department, Cyprus University of Technology, Limassol, Cyprus

University of Turku, Turku, Finland
e-mail: andreas.charalambous@cut.ac.cy

© Springer Nature Switzerland AG 2020
A. Charalambous (ed.), *Developing and Utilizing Digital Technology in Healthcare for Assessment and Monitoring*,
https://doi.org/10.1007/978-3-030-60697-8_2

an approach that best fits a "customisation" approach rather than a "personalised" or "person-centred" one. This is partly due to using the terms interchangeably when, in fact, they have different meanings and implications. Adding to the discussion is the apparent different perspectives of "individualisation" held by those in healthcare (i.e. also called as person-centred care or individualised care) and those in technology. Below a conceptual approach is provided to accommodate both views raising the commonalities as well as the discrepancies between and within the two disciplines.

Personalisation and Customisation in Technology

Personalisation as a process entails the tailoring of a service or a product to accommodate specific individuals, sometimes tied to groups or segments of individuals. When referring to personalised content, in particular, it is content that is targeted to the consumer, adaptable to each consumer's profile (i.e. usually based on specific information provided by the user or information retrieved by software according to the user's behaviour). In this context it has also been described as a means of meeting the customer's needs more effectively and efficiently, making interactions faster and easier and, consequently, increasing customer satisfaction. It is achieved when a system tailors an experience based on a consumer's previous behaviours. The conceptualisation of personalisation within the technological context is presented with an obvious weakness in capturing a true person-centred perspective. As explained above the fact that the personalisation is based on the user's previous behaviour there is a gap in between behaviour. So any technological intervention is unable to capture and adjust changes in the status of the user that might also reflect an alternative behaviour. Despite the utilisation of widely available machine learning software, these rely on a pattern demonstrated with a user's behaviour. Therefore, the ability of such programs to capture constant shifting in a person's health status (e.g. experiencing a cluster of symptoms) might lead to the expression of deviating and constant changing behaviours from "normal", limiting the ability of the technology to provide a personalised experience.

Customisation, by definition, is the action (by a user) of modifying something to suit a particular individual or task. Although brands and businesses will attempt to influence consumer decisions or try and encourage certain choices, customisation gives ultimate power to the end user. The customisation process provides obvious advantages compared to personalisation as has been defined earlier. Mainly the provision of the appropriate tool to the patient and the possibility for making adjustments to suit his/her needs seem to be the prevailing factors. However, the success of any customisation process will heavily depend on the quality of the original tool that will be provided (e.g. adaptability, responsiveness to patient's needs).

Although at a glance these two definitions appear similar, they hold a pivotal difference that lies with who is making the changes and handling this to the user is an obvious advantage to be considered. Users customise products or services to fit their own needs. Great companies personalise their products, services and communications for a user. The path by which personalisation can be achieved is mainly through the use of customer data and predictive technology. Nevertheless, the path in customisation is different as this is achieved when the user manually makes changes (to an existing product/service) to achieve his or her preferred experience. The conceptualisation of personalisation and customisation concept within the field of technology raises the question whether these concepts can be transferrable as single concepts in healthcare. In an ideal way the elements of the two processes need to be combined to better support a patient-centred approach to emerging technologies. For example a system that is initially built according to big data (e.g. available from large-scale studies) can provide a preliminary level of personalisation that could be in time further individualised based on information provided (and controlled) by the user. The constant flow of information to the technology can provide constant adjustments to real-life changes that ultimately correspond to what the user (i.e. patient) needs.

Patient-Centred Care, Personalised and Individualised Care in Healthcare

Patient-centred care (PCC) has emerged as a primary approach to healthcare. This approach emphasises partnerships in health between patients and healthcare professionals, acknowledges patients' preferences and values, promotes flexibility in the provision of healthcare and seeks to move beyond the traditional paternalistic approach to healthcare. Thus, in addition to the physical aspects of healthcare, the PCC approach acknowledges a patient's beliefs and values towards well-being [1]. PCC has also been defined as "providing care that is respectful of and responsive to individual patient preferences, needs, and values and ensuring that patient values guide all clinical decisions" [2]. Individualised nursing care, a form of person-centred care delivery, has been defined as care that has been tailored to a patient's experiences (including events associated with illness, home, work and leisure), behaviours (including physical indicators and preferred coping strategies), feelings and perceptions (including meanings ascribed to experiences and interpretations of events) [3]. Although it is safe to argue that these terms are not identical they do convey the idea that the care provided takes into consideration individuals' needs, desires, experiences, preferences, behaviours, feelings, perceptions and understandings [4].

Philosophical Underpinnings

The term person-centred care has its origins in the work of Carl Rogers, which focused on individual personal experience as the basis and standard for living and therapeutic effect [5]. Roger's person-centred approach is based on the principles and values of acceptance, caring, empathy and sensitivity in human interactions [6]. Tom Kitwood first used the term in 1988 to distinguish a certain type of care approach from more medical and behavioural approaches to dementia [7]. Essential to this and other theories on person-centred care is the providers' ability to communicate and interact with the patient in a person-centred way. For example, Kitwood used the term to bring together ideas and ways of working that emphasised communication and relationships. Caring, supported by the philosophy of humanism, grounds a person-centred approach to nursing. Humanism is defined as a doctrine, attitude, or way of life centred on human interests or values [8]. Humanistic approaches assume that individuals are capable of giving meaning to circumstances that occur in their life and are able to make decisions based on those meanings [9]. In other words, the humanistic self positions individuals to be free to make choices in their lives. The lens of humanism allows nurses to see people as holistic beings whose health is not the result of a sentinel event but, instead, the outcome of the biological, psychological and social aspects of their life experience. This view fosters in us a desire to care for individual people instead of leaving us to remain focused only on a medical disease or a curative approach.

Patient and Public Involvement in Healthcare

Developing a patient and public focus to healthcare is not a new concept and has been a long recognised area of focus within policy. It was as early as the beginning of the twenty-first century that across the world (e.g. UK, North America, Canada and Australia) this topic has become a priority in the political agenda and one that was promoted by international health organisations (e.g. WHO) as an essential component for the provision of quality care by healthcare systems. Involvement is framed as positive for individuals, the health system, public health, as well as for communities and society as a whole [10]. Patients' contribution lies in their lived experience, which may offer unique insight into healthcare service experiences, how these services affect their health, how services support them to take control of their own health, and systemic and geographical barriers to healthcare access [11]. In specific areas of healthcare their contribution though patient engagement, such as research for example, is a more straightforward and structured process that involves meaningful and active collaboration between researchers and patients in governance, priority setting, research conduct and knowledge translation.

Traditionally, models and frameworks of involvement have been defined and distinguished by the degree of power and level of involvement of patients and carers

[12]. Depending on the context that patient engagement is generated and supported there needs to be an appropriate model and framework to reflect the specificities of the occasion. Applying the appropriate model or framework is essential as each of these involvement models stem from quite distinct ideological drivers (e.g. experiential knowledge, socio-democratic drivers) and result in different ideas about auctioning them. The models and frameworks are the means that can contribute to the development of knowledge through systematic description of a phenomenon. Within the context of patient engagement, models and frameworks provide a comprehensive understanding of the core elements that underlie patient engagement, which potentially include the relationships among and flow of information between the relevant stakeholders [13].

Within the context of technology in the field of health, patient engagement can be influenced by two ideological drivers, namely Experiential knowledge and Emancipation and Empowerment. Due to the nature of the technological development within this context, patient engagement extends to include an individual's involvement in his or her own personal healthcare (e.g. decision-making and self-management) but also the involvement of the individual in research (e.g. rigorous testing of the technological intervention). The former is underpinned by the involvement of patients as partners alongside professionals in care practice and the latter has been driven by agendas underpinned by ideologies of emancipation through recognition of differential experiences of truth.

Providing a Person-Centred Experience to Technological Solutions: Reality or Fiction?

There are many challenges to technologically meet all users' needs and requirements regarding accessibility, usability, safety and acceptability along the development process of a technological solution (e.g. mobile Apps, patient portals). Despite the many challenges that present in relation to the personalisation of technological solutions, this can be a feasible outcome when the aspects of accessibility, usability, safety and acceptability are consistently and systematically taken into consideration within the development process. The level of successful integration of these aspects will eventually determine the level of the solution's personalisation and utilisation by the user.

The element of accessibility is a requirement for basic use of products by as many users as possible, in particular in special population groups with specific characteristics (e.g. elderly persons, persons with cognitive disabilities). The development process of any technological solution needs to take into consideration aspects that relate to its usability. Usability refers to the ease with which these products or services can be used to achieve specified goals with effectiveness, efficiency and satisfaction in a specified context of use [11, 14]. Safety refers to freedom from unacceptable risk that derives from the intended or unintended consequences of using a product [15]. Whereas the safety requirements apply to the intended user group, nowadays there is a tendency to extend the user group to all users, regardless of ability or age (e.g. including children). Within the healthcare area, many of the technological solutions do not only target the user (e.g. patient) but also the informal caregiver (i.e. family); therefore, any safety aspects need to take into consideration this wider reach of the product.

For accessibility, usability, safety and acceptability to have a meaningful impact, these should be taken into account during the product design ideally from early stages, following a more interactive and iterative design-development-testing procedure. There are subsequent challenges for this to be effectively applied, the major one being the cost. For example, within the context of Ambient Intelligence (AmI) solutions, the global cost of the design and development process can be critically increased since these solutions need to involve complex features such as ubiquity, context awareness, smartness, adaptiveness and computing embedded in daily life goods [16, 17].

To place the discussion in the perspective of a contextual framework we draw on the theoretical perspectives of the Technology and Acceptance Model (TAM). TAM is considered one of the most influential theories for understanding a user's acceptance and usability of emerging technologies [18]. TAM has been successfully applied to lots of research domains (e.g. various user populations and contexts) and related applications (e.g. IOT—internet of things, social gaming) and proven its capacity and validity in explaining user behaviour towards adoption of information systems [19]. To simply demonstrate how the model facilitates the acceptability and usability of emerging technologies simply consider the following example. An older adult who perceives digital games as too difficult to play or a waste of time will be unlikely to want to adopt this technology, while an older adult who perceives digital games as providing needed mental stimulation and as easy to learn will be more likely to want to learn how to use digital games [20].

The Technology and Acceptance Model posits that a person's intent to use (acceptance of technology) and usage behaviour (actual use) of a technology are predicated by the person's perceptions of the specific technology's usefulness (benefit from using the technology) and ease of use. Simply, users are more likely to adopt a new technology with high-quality UI (user interface) and UX (user experience) design (i.e., usable, useful, desirable and credible). The TAM also suggests that perceptions of usefulness and ease of use that drive a user's motivation are mediated by external variables including individual differences, system characteristics (e.g. system features, capabilities), social influences and facilitating conditions [21]. It is further suggested that user motivation consists of three influential factors, that is, perceived ease of use (PEOU), perceived usefulness (PU) and attitude towards using (ATT). The attitude towards using, which is influenced by perceived usefulness (PU) and perceived ease of use (PEOU), is the major determinant for a user to accept or reject a certain emerging technology. According to TAM, perceived usefulness (PU) and perceived ease of use (PEOU) are the most important beliefs for a user to make a decision of whether to accept the system or not [22, 23]. Within the healthcare context, the theoretical perspectives introduced by the TAM need to be incorporated within the patients' perspectives on PCC as a means to achieving optimisation of the emerging technologies' personalised profile that will facilitate their acceptance and utilisation by the patients. Despite the potential of emerging in healthcare, the aim is (or should be) synergy with humans in healthcare, rather than replacement. Within the context of Artificial Intelligence (AI) for example, in the transitional phase, validation and verification of AI algorithms is of paramount importance, while simultaneously bridging the educational gap for healthcare professionals who may not have a good understanding of AI or readily accept its implementation [24, 25]. By gradually offsetting functions that machines do best and combining these with tasks best suited for humans, this process can create and enhance a hybrid workforce. Therefore, the following eight dimensions need to be considered and incorporated within the TAM: (a) patients' preferences, (b) information and education, (c) access to care, (d) emotional support, (e) family and friends, (f) continuity and transition, (g) physical comfort and (h) coordination of care [26, 27]. These eight dimensions emphasise the fact that any efforts to develop personalised technological solutions must be designed around a deep understanding of what happens at the ground level across the patient pathway [28]. The process of incorporating patient preferences needs to be focusing on such things as shared decision-making, definition of appointments, delays and self-management, all of which are elements of an organisational approach. The establishment of (ongoing) feedback pathways will provide the patients the platform to comment and promote on the further adjustment of the technological solutions that will echo changes in the patient's status that often create a shift in his or her needs.

Conclusion

Healthcare is rapidly shifting towards a digitised future where technological solutions will prevail within the care of patients across the care continuum and across settings. However the future that is shaping in healthcare should be about the patient and the efforts to provide high-quality care in the way and in the areas that the patient prefers. The only way to achieve this is to remain committed in such a way that the delivery system designs need to be customised for each individual patient, instead of "one size fits all". The task presents with many challenges that require taking into consideration the preferences as well as the personal characteristics of the user and be able to adjust these accordingly as the user's conditions changes.

References

1. Lori JD. Patient-centred care as an approach to improving health care in Australia. Collegian. 2018;25(1):119–23.

2. Institute of Medicine. Crossing the quality chasm: a new health system for the 21st century. Washington, DC: National Academies Press; 2001.
3. Radwin LE, Alster K. Individualized nursing care: an empirically generated definition. Int Nurs Rev. 2002;49:54–63.
4. Charalambous A, Chappell NL, Katajisto J, Suhonen R. The conceptualization and measurement of individualized care. Geriatr Nurs. 2012;33(1):17–27.
5. Fazio S, Pace D, Flinner J, Kallmyer B. The Fundamentals of Person-Centered Care for Individuals With Dementia. The Gerontologist. 2018;58(1):S10–S19.
6. Rogers CR. A way of being. New York, NY: Houghton Mifflin Company; 1980.
7. Kitwood T. Toward a theory of dementia care: ethics and interaction. J Clin Ethics. 1988;9:23–34.
8. Humanism. Merriam-Webster.com Dictionary, Merriam-Webster. https://www.merriam-webster.com/dictionary/humanism. Accessed 14 Feb 2020.
9. Cheshire C, Antin J, Cook KS, Churchill E. General and familiar trust in websites. Knowl Technol Policy. 2010;23(3–4):311–31.
10. Fredriksson M, Eriksson M, Tritter J. Who wants to be involved in health care decisions? Comparing preferences for individual and collective involvement in England and Sweden. BMC Public Health. 2018;18:18.
11. Snow ME, Tweedie K, Pederson A. Heard and valued: the development of a model to meaningfully engage marginalized populations in health services planning. BMC Health Serv Res. 2018;18:181.
12. Forbat L, Hubbard G, Kearney N. Patient and public involvement: models and muddles. J Clin Nurs. 2018;18:2547–54.
13. Chudyk AM, Waldman C, Horrill T, et al. Models and frameworks of patient engagement in health services research: a scoping review protocol. Res Involv Engag. 2018;4:28.
14. Wegge KP, Zimmermann D. Accessibility, usability, safety, ergonomics: concepts, models, and differences. In: Stephanidis C, editor. Universal Access in Human Computer Interaction. Coping with Diversity. Paper presented at the 4th International Conference on Universal Access in Human-Computer Interaction, UAHCI 200, Beijing. Berlin: Springer; 2007. p. 294–301.
15. ISO/IEC. Guide 51. Safety aspects - guidelines for their inclusion in standards. Geneva: International Organization for Standardization; 1999.
16. Acampora G, Cook DJ, Rashidi P, Vasilakos AV. A survey on ambient intelligence in health care. Proc IEEE Inst Electr Electron Eng. 2013;101(12):2470–94.
17. Streitz N, Charitos D, Kaptein M, Böhlen M. Grand challenges for ambient intelligence and implications for design contexts and smart societies. J Amb Intell Smart Environ. 2019;11(1):87–107.
18. Lee Y, Kozar KA, Larsen KRT. The technology acceptance model: past, present, and future. Commun Assoc Inf Syst. 2003;12(1):752–80.
19. Chen H, Rong W, Ma X, Qu Y, Xiong Z. An extended technology acceptance model for mobile social gaming service popularity analysis. Mob Inf Syst. 2017;2017:3906953. pp 1–12.
20. Charness N, Boot WR. Technology, gaming, and social networking. In: Warner Schaie K, Willis SL, editors. Handbook of the psychology of aging. 8th ed. London: Elsevier Inc; 2016. p. 389–404.
21. Portz JD, Bayliss EA, Bull S, Boxer RS, Bekelman DB, Gleason K, Czaja S. Using the technology acceptance model to explore user experience, intent to use, and use behavior of a patient portal among older adults with multiple chronic conditions: descriptive qualitative study. J Med Internet Res. 2019;21(4):e11604.
22. Davis FD. Perceived usefulness, perceived ease of use, and user acceptance of information technology. MIS Q. 1989;13(3):319–40.
23. He Y, Chen Q, Kitkuakul S. Regulatory focus and technology acceptance: perceived ease of use and usefulness as efficacy. Cogent Bus Manag. 2018;5:1.
24. Wong NC, Shayegan B. Patient centered care for prostate cancer-how can artificial intelligence and machine learning help make the right decision for the right patient? Ann Transl Med. 2019;7(Suppl 1):S1.

25. Barrett M, Boyne J, Brandts J, et al. Artificial intelligence supported patient self-care in chronic heart failure: a paradigm shift from reactive to predictive, preventive and personalised care. EPMA J. 2019;10(4):445–64.
26. Berghout M, van Exel J, Leensvaart L, Cramm JM. Healthcare professionals' views on patient-centered care in hospitals. BMC Health Serv Res. 2015;15:385.
27. den Boer J, Nieboer AP, Cramm JM. A cross-sectional study investigating patient-centred care, co-creation of care, well-being and job satisfaction among nurses. J Nurs Manag. 2017;25(7):577–84.
28. Etienne M. Toward customized care comment on (Re) making the procrustean bed? Standardization and customization as competing logics in healthcare. Int J Health Policy Manag. 2018;7(3):272–4.

Can a Robot Provide the Answer? Ethical Considerations in Using Social Robots for Assessment and Monitoring in Healthcare

Heike Felzmann

Introduction

Social robots are increasingly entering areas of healthcare that were long considered to be essentially reliant on interpersonal interaction. According to Hegel et al. [1] "social robots were explicitly developed for the interaction of humans and robots to support a human-like interaction" (p. 170). In order to engage in social interaction, social robots have to be "able to express and perceive emotions, communicate with high-level dialogue, learn and recognize models of other agents … [and have] to be capable of establishing and maintaining social relationships" (p. 170). Social robots in healthcare are designed to complete specific care delivery tasks, partly by means of interaction with healthcare recipients and/or healthcare staff.

Social robots in healthcare have been promoted as a solution to societal challenges in providing quality care to demographics in need of specialist or particularly intense care delivery. It has been frequently highlighted that due to demographic developments in aging societies in the developed world, healthcare systems not only have increasing absolute numbers of persons in need of care, but also decreasing proportions of available healthcare professionals and carers relative to persons in need of care [2]. An important part of healthcare delivery is the need to assess and monitor patients' health state and to monitor their trajectory of recovery, maintenance or deterioration. While most social robots in healthcare are not currently at levels of autonomy and interactional complexity that would allow them to fulfil the desired functions reliably in natural settings yet, they may become a reality in the not too distant future, especially in light of substantial recent advances in artificial intelligence. Therefore, it is essential to consider the ethical considerations

H. Felzmann (✉)
School of History and Philosophy, NUI Galway, Galway, Ireland
e-mail: heike.felzmann@nuigalway.ie

© Springer Nature Switzerland AG 2020
A. Charalambous (ed.), *Developing and Utilizing Digital Technology in Healthcare for Assessment and Monitoring*,
https://doi.org/10.1007/978-3-030-60697-8_3

associated with their intended uses in healthcare settings so that planning for their introduction into real-life settings can proactively address potential problems that may arise.

Social Robots for Assessment and Monitoring

Healthcare robots have been developed for contexts as diverse as operation rooms, rehabilitation, residential and domestic care, performing robotic surgery, assisted walking, lifting, behavioural monitoring, instruction, companionship and facilitating conversation. Many healthcare robots may have assessment and monitoring functions without being social robots, such as exoskeletons which might be used for both the assessment and rehabilitation of movement impairments [3, 4]. In this chapter the focus will be specifically on social robots, with a focus on the distinctive challenges arising from the combination of social functions in assessment and monitoring. Three groups of social robots that are used for assessment and monitoring functions will be distinguished: telepresence, testing and surveillance robots.

Telepresence Robots: Personal Interaction with Remote Healthcare Professionals

One of the traditional types of social robots for assessment and monitoring purposes is telepresence robots. These are generally mobile robotic devices which serve as a means of remote communication, usually with an incorporated camera and screen that allows two-way remote communication between a healthcare professional and a patient [5]. While many telepresence robots might be described simply as "an iPad on a stick with wheels" (https://www.telepresencerobots.com/robots/double-2, 0:54/2:17), others are designed with more comprehensive social or emotional features. Some telepresence robots include physical design features that evoke social responses in recipients, such as the incorporation of facial features or anthropomorphic or zoomorphic shapes (e.g. Padbot https://www.padbot.com/index or Sanbot https://www.sanbot.co.uk/#sanbot-robot telepresence products). Those robots may also have verbal or non-verbal interactive capabilities that allow the user to engage emotionally or conversationally with the robot itself, rather than just with the remote person represented on the screen.

These devices are often used in hospital or other healthcare settings, where the mobile robot might move between patients to communicate with a remote healthcare professional who can conduct a health assessment via the robot, for example, if a specialist from another city or institution reviews a patient or if their usual care provider is only available remotely. Another common use setting is domestic care, where healthcare staff may use the telepresence robot for assessment and ongoing monitoring of a person with healthcare needs, for example in the area of care for older persons. For example, GiraffPlus (https://www.telepresencerobots.com/robots/giraff-telepresence) is a mobile telepresence healthcare robot that was developed specifically for the care of older persons in domestic settings who can live independently but are in need of slightly higher levels of care [6].

Testing Robots: Eliciting and Processing Patient Responses

Another way of performing assessment and monitoring through social robots is through offering testing that requires direct robot-patient interaction. With this class of robots, the assessment activities are initiated and performed by the robot, but depending on the capabilities of the patient the interaction may be facilitated by additional parties such as healthcare professionals or family members. While in the field of neurorehabilitation wearable robotic devices, such as exoskeletons, have long been used to assess the patients' condition through direct physical interaction with the robot of the body parts in question [3, 4], in the field of social robotics such assessment is completed through social interaction that actively elicits information from the user. Robots in this group tend to be designed specifically as socially appealing and engaging robots, often with humanoid and facial features and voice interaction that make it easy for patients to feel they are interacting with a socially responsive entity, to facilitate the engagement needed for the completion of assessment activities. For example, the humanoid care robot MARIO (http://www.mario-project.eu/portal/) included a module that allowed to complete parts of the Comprehensive Geriatric Assessment (CGA) through robot-human interaction [7, 8]. The humanoid social robot Pepper (https://www.softbankrobotics.com/emea/en/pepper) has similarly been used to perform cognitive testing of patients [9, 10]. The humanoid robot NAO (https://www.softbankrobotics.com/emea/en/nao) is frequently used for educational activities for children with autism, but it has also been used to diagnose autism-specific features in attention and behaviour in response to robot-delivered tasks [11–13]. The same robot has also been used for structured monitoring of frailty on the basis of a combination between robot-implemented questionnaire and activity tasks [14]. Similarly, the humanoid robot Zeno (https://www.hansonrobotics.com/zeno/) has been used for assessment of autism on the basis of imitation movement patterns [15].

Surveillance Robots: Robots as Windows into People's Everyday Life and Behaviour

Assessment and monitoring by social robots might also occur on the basis of continuous real-life data capture. This might rely on video, audio or other data capture representing aspects of persons' natural behaviour, but it could also combine with users' direct engagement with the robot. Especially with the substantial increase in

AI capabilities, there is significant potential for using a combination of environmental sensors with a mobile robot for collection and interpretation of data from natural settings, such as activities of daily living, activity levels, posture or emotions [16, 17]. Robots can be used as straightforward remote observation tools, allowing the observation of a person in their home or room through cameras. Other assessments may be based on the user's handling of the robot itself, as for example in the case of sensor-equipped baby robots, such as the RealCare Baby Infant Simulator (https://www.realityworks.com/product/realcare-baby-3-infant-simulator/). This robot baby tracks various parameters that are understood as indicators of safe parenting [18]. In more complex systems, the robot can be supplemented by a more comprehensive sensor network and/or complex AI to identify important parameters of a person's daily life. For example, the eWare project combines the social robot Tessa from Tinybots (https://www.tinybots.nl/) with AI to provide "lifestyle monitoring", in the sense of providing "insight into the short- and long-term life patterns of a person with dementia" (http://www.aal-europe.eu/projects/eware/, also [19]). The LARES system similarly combines a wireless sensor network and an autonomous robot [20].

Ethical Challenges

The use of social robots for such assessment and monitoring purposes is highly ethically sensitive. In this section three groups of core ethical concerns will be proposed as particularly significant for understanding the ethical challenges in using social robots for assessment and monitoring. These will then be applied to three prototypical use cases, one for each of the previously identified robot types.

Values for Assessment and Monitoring Robots

In this section, the core ethical considerations are grouped into three categories: (1) values related to assessment and monitoring, specifically assessment quality and privacy, (2) values related to the social aspects of the robots' functioning, specifically acceptability and honesty, and finally (3) the value of care in context, including stakeholder and societal considerations about care.

Values Regarding Assessment and Monitoring

Core values relating to assessment and monitoring include achieving a good quality of the assessment and privacy. A high quality of assessment and monitoring is closely linked to the ability to achieve fundamental goals of healthcare: benefitting and not harming the health of the patient. An accurate and valid assessment process is the starting point of care planning and ongoing care adjustments. Different potential deficiencies to the quality of assessment might be present, including lack of validity (the assessment does not really measure what it purports to measure) and lack of reliability and accuracy (the assessment cannot be trusted to measure what it is meant to measure in exactly the same way if repeated). Healthcare planning following a deficient assessment builds may be harmful for the patient due to misunderstanding their health state and care needs. Accordingly, it is essential that robot assessment and monitoring is carefully designed to ensure validity and accuracy.

Privacy is another core value associated with assessment and monitoring. Assessment and monitoring in healthcare are based on gathering and evaluating sensitive personal information about a person's health and well-being. If social robots collect such sensitive information on patients, it is essential that it is managed in a privacy preserving manner [21]. Privacy is a hugely complex concept, and many important dimensions of privacy are captured in data protection legislation, such as the legal framework of the European General Data Protection Regulation (GDPR). Important data-related aspects of privacy for social robots include the security and minimisation of the personal data captured. With regard to the subjective experience of privacy in assessment and monitoring by robots, the reduction of intrusiveness into what users and other stakeholders perceive as their private sphere is essential. And finally, data collection must proceed transparently, so that the user knows what information is being captured, and users' consent is ensured [21, 22].

Values Regarding Social Interaction with Robots

The social dimension of human-robot interaction is the second group of values that deserve ethical attention. Being engaged in assessment and monitoring with social robots needs to be experienced as acceptable by patient users. Acceptability is supported when robots are emotionally relatable and tap into our automatic social reactions to verbal or non-verbal clues [23]. Acceptability is threatened if users feel that the human-robot interaction is frequently disrupted or inadequate to their needs, or that they cannot communicate what they want to communicate. Users may also feel that they are treated disrespectfully when care is provided that relies on robots rather than human beings. In addition to immediate emotional responses to the robot and the experience of engaging with it, acceptability may also be linked to users' wider value perspectives on what they consider an appropriate role for a robot. For example, they may find a robot socially engaging if employed in some settings (e.g. as toy) but may experience the same or similar robots as profoundly off-putting if the robot is employed for purposes that they do not agree with (e.g. as companion for persons with dementia) [24]. Associated with this is also the concern regarding infantilisation, of users engaging in a relationship with robots that bystanders might perceive as undignified or humiliating [25].

A further important ethical aspect regarding the social experience of human-robot interaction is related to transparency or honesty. It has been argued that robots should not be deceiving users by presenting themselves as something that they are not, e.g. as animals like the seal-shaped Paro (http://www.parorobots.com/), as babies rather than inanimate dolls, or as supportive friends rather than machines [25]. In the case of social robots, one particular concern is that affective design for acceptability increases the emotional attachment of users to these robots. Especially with a highly articulate, non-verbally expressive, or emotionally responsive robot users may erroneously be led to understand their relationship to the robot as genuine and mutual. Therefore, transparency about the nature and limitations of the robot as interaction partner can be considered an important part of honest design.

Values Regarding the Realisation of Care

Care ethics has established the importance of care as ethical concept, especially for the field of healthcare. Care ethics relies on an appreciation of the importance of vulnerability and dependency in human life, and on a relational understanding of caring activities [26]. Reflections on care as an ethical concept are frequently addressed in healthcare ethics [27]. The use of robots may impact on how care is delivered and experienced by patient users. A core question regarding the value of care is how the specific use of the robotic technology impacts on care delivery, and whether it may undercut, preserve or enhance care delivery. Van Wynsberghe's [28, 29] analysis is focusing specifically on the potential contributions of robots to disrupt or support human caring. With regard to assessment and monitoring, this means that it needs to be considered whether robot-facilitated assessment or monitoring will facilitate better or worse care overall. One particularly significant concern in this context is what is sometimes called the "dehumanisation" of care [30, 31]: the risk of reduction and replacement of human contact in robot-assisted care delivery. It is important to consider that robot use does not just impact on the patient, but also on carers and family members, and also more widely on perceptions of caring responsibilities within society.

Case Examples

In order to illustrate how these values may apply to different assessment and monitoring robots a set of use cases based on the initial typology will be described and analysed with regard to their ethical challenges.

Telepresence Robots for Remote Healthcare Assessment in Hospitals

In the case of telepresence robots for remote healthcare assessment the accuracy of the assessment primarily depends on the professional competence of the healthcare professional rather than the robot itself. The contribution of the robot is primarily instrumental and facilitative and consists in providing the conditions for accurate diagnosis, such as a reliable connection that allows information to be transmitted at a sufficient level of quality [5]. Typical challenges consist in lack of access to Wifi or general internet connectivity in the hospital setting, unsuitable ambient conditions for the sensors available (e.g. due to low lighting or high ambient noise), or insufficient flexibility of the robot to adjust to specific information requirements of the patient or professional. These might lead to a misdiagnosis or inaccurate communication between patient and healthcare professional. It is therefore essential to ensure that accurate diagnosis and effective communication are possible under the likely deployment conditions, requiring potentially extended context-specific testing [5].

Regarding privacy, telepresence robots that are used for communications between the healthcare provider and the patient generally are made clearly aware when the telepresence begins and ends and who is connected to them. Some systems are also designed in a way that their camera automatically faces the wall when not in use [5]. Under such conditions, there are low levels of intrusiveness, and the users are aware of information being shared if they have to activate the robot for incoming calls. It would, however, need to be clarified to them what, if any, information beyond the live communication is being shared with the remote professional or stored on the device. For example, the original GiraffPlus robot had a number of integrated sensors for assessment beyond mere facilitation of communication [6]. Respecting privacy would require that any use of information beyond the overt live communication is flagged to users and actively consented for.

With regard to acceptability and user engagement, in telepresence robots the primary interactive engagement of the patient is with the remote healthcare professional, not the robot itself. For the "iPad on a stick with wheels" robot, few additional emotionally engaging aspects are included, apart from the communication interface. For morphologically more emotionally appealing telepresence robots, such as robots with humanoid or zoomorphic shape, the design of the robot might contribute to further positive predisposition to engage with the robot-facilitated communication [32]. Acceptability will be dependent on whether users accept remote interaction as sufficiently satisfactory for their needs; indications are that users often accept remote interaction as a satisfactory replacement [33].

In general, telepresence robots can be considered as transparent with regard to their function and the nature of the robot. The simple versions of these robots present themselves clearly as a communicative tool that facilitates communication, and not as a communicative agent in its own right. However, this boundary becomes more blurred when facilitating telepresence is just one among many functions of the robot, and the robot also communicates directly with the user, for example for the performance of assistive or companionship functions. In those cases, more care needs to be taken to achieve transparency regarding the robot's functions and limitations.

From the perspective of the value of care, it needs to be considered how facilitating remote communication with healthcare professionals contributes to care delivery. This depends strongly on the wider context of their use. On the one hand, telepresence can be identified as a helpful tool to facilitate communication when face-to-face presence of the healthcare professional is not feasible, due to physical or time restrictions. For example, a larger team may be enabled to consult with a patient without causing disruption to the unit through entry of a number of professionals at the same time [5]. It may also allow access to expertise that might otherwise not be available in the location. It may facilitate continuity of care with the same professional and thereby allow the patient and the professional to build up a better relationship [33]. All these have been identified in studies on telepresence robots as potential benefits for the patient and care providers. However, technical limitations of remote communication, lack of non-verbal signs, and the lack of human touch and bodily presence may also negatively affect the experience of the quality of care. From a wider care delivery system perspective, normalisation of remote communication may lead to increasing replacement of face-to-face communication which would be potentially problematic. This might be exacerbated if telepresence robots also become a primary means of communication with family members and other social contacts. How exactly the longer term use of these robots will impact on the care experience therefore needs to be followed up through careful investigation of the care experience by patients and professional users; existing studies for situations where remote interaction still was the exception may not be applicable to contexts in which they have become normalised or even a dominant mode of communication.

Robot-Facilitated Testing of Children with Autism

Social robots for persons with autism are sometimes designed to provide a combination of assessment and training. Robots might assess the presence of features indicative of autism, such as deficits in gesture imitation, joint attention or communication [11, 12, 15], while also providing educational interventions. There is a comprehensive body of research on the use of robots with persons with autism which has shown that the willingness to engage with robots appears to be comparatively high among children with autism [34].

In relation to the quality of assessment, some robot-assessed features of autism-specific parameters, such as gaze direction for joint attention, can be measured by robot sensors with high accuracy [12]. In contrast, for other important features such as the adequacy of interpersonal communication robots may only be able to assess certain aspects and results may still require interpretation by human assessors. From a quality of assessment perspective, for a condition that is as multifaceted and complex as autism and presents in such an individualised manner it is crucial that no oversimplification occurs in the process of assessment. It might be tempting to focus assessment around parameters that are particularly easily implemented by the robot. However, if the assessment is linked to interventions, it needs to provide a practical basis for intervention planning, and the interventions performed must be those that are most meaningful for the life of the person with autism.

Privacy challenges arise especially with regard to the lack of transparency of assessment, especially if assessment tasks are presented in a playful manner or resemble educational interventions. A core principle of privacy is giving persons control over their personal information by requiring consent; in the case of children, a combination of parental consent and child assent is desirable if feasible. Apart from transparency and consent, data security for the personal data collected by the robot is also essential, especially if recognisable information such as video is being collected. The requirement of data minimisation is also pertinent, especially if large amounts of data are being captured and more complex parameters are being assessed, as would be required if the robot is designed to perform automated assessment of complex characteristics. It is essential to consider whether the benefit from such assessment outweighs the associated data protection risks. Interestingly, a study of stakeholder attitudes on autism robots did not show existence of major concerns for privacy and data protection, but as the study's authors pointed out, this might have been due to a lack of awareness of data processing in robots rather than the ethical irrelevance of these considerations [35].

As already indicated, robots have been shown to be acceptable and engaging for children with autism, provided their design features match their processing characteristics [36]. It has been argued that for this target group the lower complexity of social cues and absence of distractive social features of robots may allow children to benefit more easily from the interaction with robots compared with human interaction. However, careful user studies are needed to ensure that this is indeed the case and not just the result of stereotyping of persons with ASD.

Testing through robots should be clearly presented as such, to meet the requirement of honesty and transparency. Especially when assessment and play or education are combined and when the robot is designed to be appealing to the user, the purpose of assessment may become easily obscured and should be explicitly presented to the user.

Using robot-supported assessment as part of the care for children with autism requires careful attention to the use of the robot within the care process. It has been argued that testing for autism is a protracted and potentially unpleasant process and that therefore the child and professionals may benefit from letting robots take on some of the time-consuming and tedious assessment tasks [13]. This appears to be in keeping with a study that looked into the acceptability of autism robots for various societal stakeholders, including the question of their use for diagnosis and progress monitoring, which showed that the majority of respondents was in favour of this type of use [37]. However, it would be essential to continue capturing professionals', patients' and family members' views on how the use of robots for these purposes affects the nature of care delivery. Concerns around wider societal acceptability of giving robots an extended role in the care provision for vulnerable persons with autism were apparent in the answers by stakeholders in this study who expressed strong preferences against the replacement of human therapists by robots, in keeping with similar concerns with regard to uses of social robots in other application domains. This would mirror care ethical concerns about societal neglect of vulnerable persons with care needs [26].

Domestic Monitoring for Older Persons or Persons with Dementia

Assistive robots are considered especially frequently for the use in domestic settings for older persons and persons with dementia, with the purpose of monitoring their safety and activities in their everyday life, e.g. potential falls, taking medication, food intake or lack of activities of daily living. Such monitoring might consist in video monitoring alone or the combination of various ambient sensors to capture users' activity remotely, for review by formal or informal carers. Increasing AI capabilities open up further possibilities for more complex analysis of information on users' activities, combing ambient networks and robots [16, 17].

Regarding the quality of assessment and monitoring significant challenges arise if the robot is not capturing relevant patient activity due to technical glitches, low-quality information streams or inadequate algorithms. For robots with a strong AI component, the correct interpretation of behaviour may be particularly challenging, especially in the context of dementia where speech behaviour patterns may be less predictable and recognisable for AI analysis. Faulty interpretation of behaviour could lead to false negatives and false positives regarding risk levels. On the one hand, lack of alarm in the case of falls or inaccurate interpretations of users' behaviour could leave patients in harm's way; on the other hand, frequent false alarms might be disruptive for all stakeholders and reduce the usefulness of the robot. Accordingly, it is essential that sensors and algorithms are carefully tested and validated under real use conditions. Another significant challenge regarding quality of assessment is the robot's usability for patients, insofar as the robot needs to allow intuitive, effortless and smooth use for older persons who may encounter the robot with a combination of dementia-related and other age-typical impairments [31].

Domestic monitoring robots are particularly ethically challenging with regard to the issue of privacy. In order to fulfil its monitoring function the robot is effectively surveilling the user by gathering data continuously about their activities within their private sphere. Privacy concerns include not just concerns about the amount and sensitivity of data collected and data security, but also a wider sense of intrusion into the private sphere. It has been pointed out that due to the level of intrusion it is particularly important that those who are being monitored see it as furthering their own goals or have some sense of control over the monitoring, in keeping with findings regarding other tracking and monitoring technologies for persons with dementia [38]. Accordingly, achieving transparency for users about the nature of the monitoring and allow some adjustments to surveillance levels is particularly important for the class of surveillance robots. This challenge has given rise to attempts to develop privacy respecting domestic technologies for older persons that nevertheless can increase their safety, such as the E.T.H.O.S. project (https://ethos.luddy.indiana.edu/).

One prominent concern regarding the acceptability of these technologies is the design of the users' engagement with the robot and with those who have access to the monitoring data. Many domestic monitoring robots are designed to fulfil also companionship and assistive functions. What makes such robots acceptable as domestic companions, especially their humanoid and affective design that fosters emotional engagement, may be problematic from the point of view of honesty and transparency, and may be even seen as a form of ethically problematic deception [39]. A robot that presents itself to the user as pleasant conversation partner not only leads to a greater level of trust, feeling of companionship and disclosure by the user [40], but may also be seen to disguise the data gathering and monitoring nature of the robot, for example, if the user is not made aware by the robot when and what data is being displayed to or accessed by carers.

The contribution of domestic monitoring robots to the realisation of care is a complex issue. On the one hand, these robots are often presented as a solution to the problem of premature institutionalisation. Staying independently in their own homes is in keeping with the wishes of many older persons, and providing continuous risk monitoring by means of a robot thereby could be seen as an appropriate adjustment of care to the needs of users, potentially benefitting users and carers by reducing care burdens without sacrificing safety and well-being. If the use of these robots, due to their telepresence functions, leads to increased time spent with remote carers, friends or loved ones, this also addresses the problem of isolation, a serious concern for many older persons with dementia [41]. It has been shown that at least under some circumstances, domestic long-term use of robots can create a positive emotional bond, especially if the robot expressions are perceived as caring and supportive [42]. However, the creation of a relationship with the robot rather than human carers could be seen as structurally problematic in the area of care of older persons with dementia, where high levels of social isolation and loneliness are very common [43] and appear to be causally connected [44, 45]. Even if human replacement of monitoring and care activities is not perceived as subjectively problematic by users whose feeling of loneliness might be alleviated by human-robot interaction, to employ a robot instead of a human for care might still be considered to exacerbate the problem of social isolation if it leads to reduction of engagement with human carers. Assistive robots are often being presented as a strategic solution to the problem of reduced societal availability of human care [2], which is ethically worrying insofar as the underlying motivation is the management of scarcity, not the development of an optimal approach to care.

In light of the ethical considerations outlined in this section, the last section focuses on the question how these ethical issues can be addressed in the design and implementation of robots for assessment and monitoring.

Value-Sensitive Design and Deployment Planning

One promising approach to the integration of ethical considerations into the design process of information technologies is value-sensitive design [46, 47]. It is a structured approach that embeds awareness of values into the design of information technologies, by engaging in an iterative design process that moves back and forth between a value analysis, the gathering of stakeholder information, and the technological side of the development. Van Wynsberghe [28, 29] has proposed an approach to value-sensitive design specifically for healthcare robots that centres around the realisation of the value of care.

With regard to social robots for monitoring and assessment, the preceding section identified some core values that such robots should be designed to realise. These included (1) values related to assessment and monitoring, specifically assessment quality and privacy, (2) values related to the social aspects of the robots' functioning, specifically acceptability and transparency, and finally (3) the value of care in context, including stakeholder and societal considerations about care. Paying explicit attention to these values in the design process can help with the proactive identification of solutions to the problems outlined in this chapter and with embedding these solutions in the robot design, for example by translating these values into specific features or functionalities.

Identifying how the use of robots can do justice to these ethical values also requires considering them when planning the robot's deployment. Envisaging ethical consequences arising from the use of technologies can be approached in various ways but requires the management of complexity and uncertainty [48–50]. Developers may see their ethical responsibilities as fulfilled once the robot has been designed, and organisations may be considered responsible for deciding how to use them. However, the interface between the development and deployment deserves more attention, as it requires both specific organisational knowledge, to do justice to their particular characteristics, but also general guidance on the conditions that need to be in place when deploying the robot. This requires substantially more than communicating technical requirements and health and safety aspects. Organisations and professionals at the coalface of care delivery cannot be expected to solve these problems without support from those who are most familiar with the robot.

One potential means of supporting such a process can be ethics checklists. While ethics checklists have received criticism across various field of ethics assessment [51], in particular the criticism that they do not do justice to the complexity of the relevant ethical considerations, their popularity across ethics domains is due to their potential to focus professionals' attention to specific ethical issues in a structured manner [52]. However, even strong proponents of ethics checklists acknowledge that sufficient space needs to be given to exploring the complexity of ethical considerations and engaging stakeholders [49].

Once ethical considerations regarding the use of the robots have been satisfactorily identified, it is essential that sufficiently robust training be provided to those using these robots. This needs to address not just the robots' specific technical functions but also how they could be used, given different circumstances, and in particular needs to identify the conditions under which the robot is likely to work in the intended manner or which conditions might prove problematic. Such training would need to include addressing considerations with regard to the three groups of values: assessment values, robot interaction values and care values. Professional users will need to understand assessment functions, how human-robot relationships are created, and be given space to explore how they can be used to contribute constructively to existing care delivery systems. The responsibility of provision of training for the professionals who will work with the robots needs to be taken on board by robot manufacturers as well by professional training bodies. If robots become an integral part of healthcare settings, healthcare professionals have to be expertly supported in working with these robots, by a combination of structured guidance and provision of opportunities to carefully reflect on the impact that these technologies might have on their professional practice.

Conclusion

As this chapter has shown, social robots can provide different types of assessment and monitoring in a variety of healthcare settings. Core ethical values relating to assessment and monitoring in care were proposed and applied to different use cases. In light of the complexity of the ethical concerns, a need was shown for taking a structured approach to the design and deployment of robots that takes seriously the need of healthcare professionals to understand these robots and be able to engage proactively with ethical challenges in their implementation.

References

1. Hegel F, Muhl C, Wrede B, Hielscher-Fastabend M, Sagerer G. Understanding social robots. In: Second International Conferences on Advances in Computer-Human Interactions 2009. Washington, DC: IEEE; 2009. p. 169–74.
2. SPARC. Robotics 2020. Multi-annual roadmap for robotics in Europe. 2016. https://www.eu-robotics.net/cms/upload/topic_groups/H2020_Robotics_Multi-Annual_Roadmap_ICT-2017B.pdf.
3. McKenzie A, Dodakian L, See J, Le V, Quinlan EB, Bridgford C, Head D, Han VL, Cramer SC. Validity of robot-based assessments of upper extremity function. Arch Phys Med Rehabil. 2017;98(10):1969–76.
4. Lambercy O, Lünenburger L, Gassert R, Bolliger M. Robots for measurement/clinical assessment. In: Neurorehabilitation technology. London: Springer; 2012. p. 443–56.
5. Kristoffersson A, Coradeschi S, Loutfi A. A review of mobile robotic telepresence. Adv Hum Comput Interact. 2013;2013:902316. https://doi.org/10.1155/2013/902316.
6. Coradeschi S, Cesta A, Cortellessa G, Coraci L, Galindo C, Gonzalez J, Karlsson L, Forsberg A, Frennert S, Furfari F, Loutfi A. GiraffPlus: a system for monitoring activities and physiological parameters and promoting social interaction for elderly. In: Human-computer systems interaction: backgrounds and applications 3. Cham: Springer; 2014. p. 261–71.
7. Asprino L, Gangemi A, Nuzzolese AG, Presutti V, Recupero DR, Russo A. Autonomous comprehensive geriatric assessment. In: AnSWeR@ ESWC 2017. p. 42–5.
8. D'onofrio G, Sancarlo D, Raciti M, Russo A, Ricciardi F, Presutti V, Messervey T, Cavallo F, Giuliani F, Greco A. MARIO project: validation in the hospital setting. In: Italian Forum of Ambient Assisted Living. Cham: Springer; 2018. p. 509–20.
9. Varrasi S, Di Nuovo S, Conti D, Di Nuovo A. A social robot for cognitive assessment. In: Companion of the 2018 ACM/IEEE International Conference on Human-Robot Interaction. Washington, DC: IEEE; 2018. p. 269–70.

10. Di Nuovo A, Varrasi S, Conti D, Bamsforth J, Lucas A, Soranzo A, McNamara J. Usability evaluation of a robotic system for cognitive testing. In: 14th ACM/IEEE International Conference on Human-Robot Interaction (HRI) 2019. Washington, DC: IEEE; 2019. p. 588–9.
11. Anzalone SM, Boucenna S, Cohen D, Chetouani M. Autism assessment through a small humanoid robot. In: Proc. HRI: A Bridge between Robotics and Neuroscience, Workshop of the 9th ACM/IEEE Int. Conf. Human-Robot Interaction. Washington, DC: IEEE; 2014. p. 1–2.
12. Anzalone SM, Xavier J, Boucenna S, Billeci L, Narzisi A, Muratori F, Cohen D, Chetouani M. Quantifying patterns of joint attention during human-robot interactions: an application for autism spectrum disorder assessment. Pattern Recogn Lett. 2019;118:42–50.
13. Petric F, Hrvatinić K, Babić A, Malovan L, Miklić D, Kovačić Z, Cepanec M, Stošić J, Šimleša S. Four tasks of a robot-assisted autism spectrum disorder diagnostic protocol: first clinical tests. In: IEEE Global Humanitarian Technology Conference (GHTC 2014). Washington, DC: IEEE; 2014. p. 510–7.
14. Keizer RA, Van Velsen L, Moncharmont M, Riche B, Ammour N, Del Signore S, Zia G, Hermens H, N'Dja A. Using socially assistive robots for monitoring and preventing frailty among older adults: a study on usability and user experience challenges. Heal Technol. 2019;9(4):595–605.
15. Wijayasinghe IB, Ranatunga I, Balakrishnan N, Bugnariu N, Popa DO. Human–robot gesture analysis for objective assessment of autism spectrum disorder. Int J Soc Robot. 2016;8(5):695–707.
16. Cook DJ, Augusto JC, Jakkula VR. Ambient intelligence: technologies, applications, and opportunities. Pervas Mob Comput. 2009;5(4):277–98.
17. Ienca M, Wangmo T, Jotterand F, Kressig RW, Elger B. Ethical design of intelligent assistive technologies for dementia: a descriptive review. Sci Eng Ethics. 2018;24(4):1035–55.
18. Søgaard VF. Forældre for en babyrobot: Et sociologisk fokus på styring af forældreskab blandt marginaliserede unge. Unpublished PhD dissertation. Aarhus University, Aarhus, DK. 2019.
19. Casaccia S, Revel GM, Scalise L, Bevilacqua R, Rossi L, Paauwe RA, Karkowsky I, Ercoli I, Serrano JA, Suijkerbuijk S, Lukkien D. Social robot and sensor network in support of activity of daily living for people with dementia. In: Dementia Lab Conference. Cham: Springer; 2019. p. 128–35.
20. Ropero F, Vaquerizo-Hdez D, Muñoz P, Barrero DF, R-Moreno MD. LARES: an AI-based teleassistance system for emergency home monitoring. Cogn Syst Res. 2019;56:213–22.
21. Kaminski ME, Rueben M, Smart WD, Grimm CM. Averting robot eyes. Maryland Law Rev. 2016;76:983–1024.
22. Vitale J, Tonkin M, Herse S, Ojha S, Clark J, Williams MA, Wang X, Judge W. Be more transparent and users will like you: a robot privacy and user experience design experiment. In: Proceedings of the 2018 ACM/IEEE International Conference on Human-Robot Interaction. Washington, DC: IEEE; 2018. p. 379–87.
23. Whelan S, Murphy K, Barrett E, Krusche C, Santorelli A, Casey D. Factors affecting the acceptability of social robots by older adults including people with dementia or cognitive impairment: a literature review. Int J Soc Robot. 2018;10(5):643–68.
24. Salvini P, Laschi C, Dario P. Design for acceptability: improving robots' coexistence in human society. Int J Soc Robot. 2010;2(4):451–60.
25. Sharkey A, Sharkey N. Granny and the robots: ethical issues in robot care for the elderly. Ethics Inf Technol. 2012;14(1):27–40.
26. Kittay EF. Love's labor: essays on women, equality and dependency. London: Routledge; 2019.
27. Tronto JC. An ethic of care. Generations. J Am Soc Aging. 1998;22(3):15–20.
28. Van Wynsberghe A. Designing robots for care: care centered value-sensitive design. Sci Eng Ethics. 2013;19(2):407–33.
29. Van Wynsberghe A. Healthcare robots: ethics, design and implementation. London: Routledge; 2016.

30. Royakkers L, van Est R. A literature review on new robotics: automation from love to war. Int J Soc Robot. 2015;7(5):549–70.
31. Wu YH, Fassert C, Rigaud AS. Designing robots for the elderly: appearance issue and beyond. Arch Gerontol Geriatr. 2012;54(1):121–6.
32. Kidd CD, Breazeal C. Effect of a robot on user perceptions. In: 2004 IEEE/RSJ International Conference on Intelligent Robots and Systems (IROS) (IEEE Cat. No. 04CH37566), vol. 4. Washington, DC: IEEE; 2004. p. 3559–64.
33. Ellison LM, Nguyen M, Fabrizio MD, Soh A, Permpongkosol S, Kavoussi LR. Postoperative robotic telerounding: a multicenter randomized assessment of patient outcomes and satisfaction. Arch Surg. 2007;142(12):1177–81.
34. Pennisi P, Tonacci A, Tartarisco G, Billeci L, Ruta L, Gangemi S, Pioggia G. Autism and social robotics: a systematic review. Autism Res. 2016;9(2):165–83.
35. Coeckelbergh M, Pop C, Simut R, Peca A, Pintea S, David D, Vanderborght B. A survey of expectations about the role of robots in robot-assisted therapy for children with ASD: ethical acceptability, trust, sociability, appearance, and attachment. Sci Eng Ethics. 2016;22(1):47–65.
36. Cabibihan JJ, Javed H, Ang M, Aljunied SM. Why robots? A survey on the roles and benefits of social robots in the therapy of children with autism. Int J Soc Robot. 2013;5(4):593–618.
37. Peca A. Robot enhanced therapy for children with autism disorders: measuring ethical acceptability. IEEE Technol Soc Mag. 2016;35(2):54–66.
38. Meiland F, Innes A, Mountain G, Robinson L, van der Roest H, García-Casal JA, Gove D, Thyrian JR, Evans S, Dröes RM, Kelly F. Technologies to support community-dwelling persons with dementia: a position paper on issues regarding development, usability, effectiveness and cost-effectiveness, deployment, and ethics. JMIR Rehabil Assist Technol. 2017;4(1):e1.
39. Matthias A. Robot lies in health care: when is deception morally permissible? Kennedy Inst Ethics J. 2015;25(2):169–92.
40. Martelaro N, Nneji VC, Ju W, Hinds P. Tell me more designing HRI to encourage more trust, disclosure, and companionship. In: 2016 11th ACM/IEEE International Conference on Human-Robot Interaction (HRI). Washington, DC: IEEE; 2016. p. 181–8.
41. Moyle W, Arnautovska U, Ownsworth T, Jones C. Potential of telepresence robots to enhance social connectedness in older adults with dementia: an integrative review of feasibility. Int Psychogeriatr. 2017;29(12):1951–64.
42. Kidd CD, Breazeal C. Robots at home: understanding long-term human-robot interaction. In: 2008 IEEE/RSJ International Conference on Intelligent Robots and Systems. Washington, DC: IEEE; 2008. p. 3230–5.
43. Moyle W, Kellett U, Ballantyne A, Gracia N. Dementia and loneliness: an Australian perspective. J Clin Nurs. 2011;20(9-10):1445–53.
44. Penninkilampi R, Casey AN, Singh MF, Brodaty H. The association between social engagement, loneliness, and risk of dementia: a systematic review and meta-analysis. J Alzheimers Dis. 2018;66(4):1619–33.
45. Rafnsson SB, Orrell M, d'Orsi E, Hogervorst E, Steptoe A. Loneliness, social integration, and incident dementia over 6 years: prospective findings from the English Longitudinal Study of Ageing. J Gerontol Ser B. 2020;75(1):114–24.
46. Friedman B, Kahn PH, Borning A. Value sensitive design and information systems. In: The handbook of information and computer ethics. Hoboken, NJ: John Wiley & Sons, Inc; 2008. p. 69–101.
47. Friedman B, Hendry DG, Borning A. A survey of value sensitive design methods. Found Trends Hum Comput Interact. 2017;11(2):63–125.
48. Brey PA. Anticipatory ethics for emerging technologies. NanoEthics. 2012;6(1):1–13.
49. Assasi N, Schwartz L, Tarride JE, Campbell K, Goeree R. Methodological guidance documents for evaluation of ethical considerations in health technology assessment: a systematic review. Exp Rev Pharmacoecon Outcomes Res. 2014;14(2):203–20.

50. Reijers W, Wright D, Brey P, Weber K, Rodrigues R, O'Sullivan D, Gordijn B. Methods for practising ethics in research and innovation: a literature review, critical analysis and recommendations. Sci Eng Ethics. 2018;24(5):1437–81.
51. Kiran AH, Oudshoorn N, Verbeek PP. Beyond checklists: toward an ethical-constructive technology assessment. J Respons Innov. 2015;2(1):5–19.
52. Nordgren A. Personal health monitoring: ethical considerations for stakeholders. J Inf Commun Ethics Soc. 2013;11(3):156–73.

Development and Implementation of Patient-Reported Outcome Measures in Cancer Care

André Manuel da Silva Lopes, Sara Colomer-Lahiguera, and Manuela Eicher

MeSH Terms: Patient-reported outcome measures; Telemedicine; Patient-centered care; Psychometrics; Neoplasms

Electronic Patient-Reported Outcomes: Definition

Patient-centered care is the hallmark of modern healthcare. At the turn of the century, focusing on the patient experience made care more effective in meeting patients' needs and is now a defining characteristic of quality care [1]. Bringing patient-reported outcomes to healthcare was one of the products of this paradigm shift.

Patient-reported outcomes (PROs) are a patient's report on the status of their own health condition, without interpretation by any third party [2]. Their use is instrumental in bringing the patient perspective into healthcare and allows clinicians to identify unmet needs and improve care. PROs can be used to assess a patient's symptoms and symptom burden, functional status, health behaviors, and health-related quality of life (HRQoL).

The need to assess PROs reliably paved the way for patient-reported outcomes measures (PROMs). A PROM is a standardized and validated instrument to measure patients' perceptions of their own well-being and health status, most often in the form of a questionnaire [2]. PROMs are often tailored to a certain health condition

A. M. da Silva Lopes · M. Eicher (✉)
Institute of Higher Education and Research in Healthcare – IUFRS, Faculty of Biology and Medicine – FBM, UNIL, Lausanne, Switzerland

Department of Oncology, Lausanne University Hospital, Lausanne, Vaud, Switzerland
e-mail: andre.da-silva-lopes@chuv.ch; manuela.eicher@chuv.ch, manuela.eicher@unil.ch

S. Colomer-Lahiguera
Institute of Higher Education and Research in Healthcare – IUFRS, Faculty of Biology and Medicine – FBM, UNIL, Lausanne, Switzerland
e-mail: sara.colomer-lahiguera@chuv.ch

© Springer Nature Switzerland AG 2020
A. Charalambous (ed.), *Developing and Utilizing Digital Technology in Healthcare for Assessment and Monitoring*,
https://doi.org/10.1007/978-3-030-60697-8_4

or disease and are used in clinical trials to assess disease activity, manage symptoms, inform treatment pathways, and support drug approval and labeling claims [2–6]. Usually these instruments are in paper form, and although this has been a practical and accessible medium, it can generate unreadable and missing data, leading to questions about their reliability in routine care [7].

Electronic patient-reported outcomes (ePROs) are essentially PROs conveyed through an electronic platform that can include interactive voice response systems (using a telephone), internet-based systems (webpages that usually collect text-based input), and device-based systems that use software applications [7]. In the same way, electronic PROMs (ePROMS) are electronic versions of the instruments that collect those outcomes. While a more significant initial investment, ePROMs overcome some of the previously mentioned worrying disadvantages of analog PROMs. The advent of widespread interconnected devices has facilitated the introduction of ePROMs in both clinical trials and routine care, as patients can use electronic devices to access questionnaires and get automated reminders that bolster adherence and completion rates. In oncology, the use of ePROMs has shown promise not just in remotely controlling symptoms and symptomatic adverse events, but also in improving overall quality of life, and even overall survival rates [8, 9].

The use of PROs has thus become a more popular goal, as it aligns itself with the benefits of e-health in oncology and a value-based model of care [10, 11]. It holds promise to enable patients to obtain better outcomes at lower costs, providers to deliver care more efficiently, while yielding better patient satisfaction. Their most valuable contribution, however, is broadening the understanding of the patient perspective. Bringing the patient closer is the means through which we achieve an important goal of modern healthcare: enable a collaborative approach to healthcare, where patients actively participate in the shared decision-making, coordination, and cooperation processes of care.

How to Develop Patient-Reported Outcome Measures

The development of PROMs has been investigated for several decades in different disciplines. Thus, the development of PROMs can be based on robust conceptual frameworks that are rooted in psychometrics on the one hand and patient-centered approaches on the other. A widely used framework that provides stepwise and iterative guidance for the development of PROMs is the FDA Guidance for Patient-Reported Outcome Measures [2]. According to this guidance, the adequacy of any PROM depends on whether its characteristics, conceptual framework, content validity, and other measurement properties are addressed sufficiently. This is valid for all PROMs, regardless of if they are measured electronically, paper based, or otherwise. The development history should be transparent and the PROM needs to be made publicly available. The minimum requirement is to describe the content validity of the PROM and this procedure should include open-ended patient input from the target population. The whole process of development is much more complex (see Fig. 1). We refer the reader to the original guidance for further details [2].

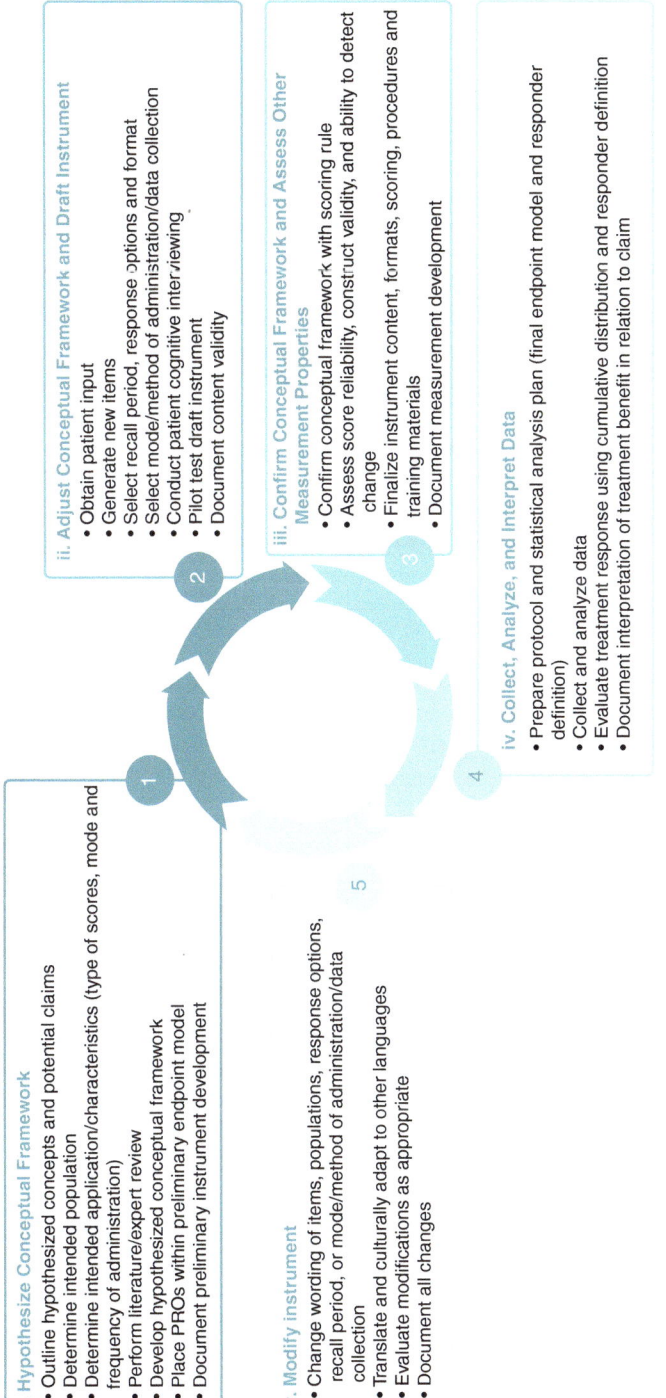

i. Hypothesize Conceptual Framework
- Outline hypothesized concepts and potential claims
- Determine intended population
- Determine intended application/characteristics (type of scores, mode and frequency of administration)
- Perform literature/expert review
- Develop hypothesized conceptual framework
- Place PROs within preliminary endpoint model
- Document preliminary instrument development

ii. Adjust Conceptual Framework and Draft Instrument
- Obtain patient input
- Generate new items
- Select recall period, response options and format
- Select mode/method of administration/data collection
- Conduct patient cognitive interviewing
- Pilot test draft instrument
- Document content validity

iii. Confirm Conceptual Framework and Assess Other Measurement Properties
- Confirm conceptual framework with scoring rule
- Assess score reliability, construct validity, and ability to detect change
- Finalize instrument content, formats, scoring, procedures and training materials
- Document measurement development

iv. Collect, Analyze, and Interpret Data
- Prepare protocol and statistical analysis plan (final endpoint model and responder definition)
- Collect and analyze data
- Evaluate treatment response using cumulative distribution and responder definition
- Document interpretation of treatment benefit in relation to claim

v. Modify instrument
- Change wording of items, populations, response options, recall period, or mode/method of administration/data collection
- Translate and culturally adapt to other languages
- Evaluate modifications as appropriate
- Document all changes

Fig. 1 Guidance for the use and development of patient-reported outcome measures in trials. (Source: U.S. Food and Drug Administration guidance for industry: patient-reported outcome measures: use in medical product development to support labeling claims. Rockville, MD: Department of Health and Human Services, Food and Drug Administration, Center for Drug Evaluation and Research; 2009, [21])

As mentioned above, ePROMs are increasingly used in clinical practice and research. Their use should nevertheless undergo several tests before they can be considered as valid and reliable, especially when they are used for research purposes. An important issue is the test of equivalence between electronic and paper-based PROMs, since available PROMs usually have been developed and tested on a paper basis. The International Society for Pharmacoeconomics and Outcomes Research (ISPOR) has published recommendations on how to investigate the measurement equivalence between electronic and paper-PROMs [12]. They recommend different levels of evidence for different levels of modification:

- Minor modifications: if no content or meaning is changed, and modifications are based on logic or existing literature (e.g., changes in instructions from circling the responses with a pen to touching the screen), cognitive debriefing/usability testing is recommended.
- Moderate modifications: if content or meaning may be change based on current empirical literature (e.g., changes in item wording) equivalence testing and usability testing are recommended.
- Substantial modifications: if content or meaning is changed without empirical support for the equivalence (e.g., substantial change in item response options or item wording) a full psychometric testing and usability testing are recommended.

With the rapid evolution of electronic health, we believe that the development of new PROMs will be increasingly based on ePROMS. The guidelines and recommendations illustrated above remain important to guarantee valid, reliable data as well as user-friendly and accepted measurements.

Implementing Electronic PROs: Opportunities and Challenges

Currently, ePROs are mainly used in the context of clinical trials, which leads to the question if they can be used in routine care, and if their benefits can make that transition as well. In countries like the Unites States, the United Kingdom, and Sweden, PROs are used to assess the quality of care and to focus quality improvement efforts, or are tied to a specific health condition to inform treatment decisions [13]. However, even in those countries both opportunities and challenges to the implementation of ePROs remain present on every level of the healthcare continuum, from the patient and provider levels to the healthcare-system level.

At the healthcare-system level, arguably the most significant opportunity for ePROs is in improving the accessibility of care for underserved communities that may have decreased access to differentiated, specialized care [14]. Enabling remote monitoring of patients can reduce the need for frequent medical visits, crossing geographical and socioeconomic barriers, while remaining a cost-effective solution, which equally benefits both rural and urban communities [4, 14, 15]. However, while ePROs can be cost-effective, their initial implementation can be prohibitively expensive: high initial costs are associated with the equipment, technical support, and professional training that are required [16].

Some of that cost has been curbed by the bring-your-own-device (BYOD) approach, where ePROs are collected using patients' own electronic devices, which have become ubiquitous [17]. This approach also introduces additional challenges related to the distribution of the software, the equivalence of the ePROM across devices (different devices may introduce slight changes in the interface of the instrument), as well as privacy and security concerns surrounding the collected data. Transparency in what data is collected and how, as well as access to it, are paramount values covered by the General Data Protection Regulation (GDPR) introduced by the European Union in 2017, which has benefited this approach [18]. In clinical trials, BYOD implies that the data is no longer under the exclusive control of the study sponsor, who is held as accountable for security and privacy breaches under the GDPR [18]. Thus, ePRO adoption can be hindered, as the requirements for lawful compliance are increasingly strict.

The aforementioned challenge is also applicable when considering the integration of ePRO data into the patient's electronic health record (EHR), arguably one of the greatest benefits of ePRO at the provider level [19]. A persistent issue in routine care is the presence of multiple sources of data that requires manual transfer and integration in the EHR. The ability to collect ePROs in real time and integrate them directly into the EHR holds the promise of making data immediately available across the care continuum, without the need for human interaction and thus minimizing transcription errors or incomplete data.

The addition of ePRO data to what is already a large volume of health data in EHRs can be a challenge in itself. The potential benefits are only as great as the quality of the data that is collected, which needs to be actionable and relevant for professionals providing care [19]. When patient assessment is already of high quality in routine care, skepticism grows on the value of that additional data, which can seem redundant [13].

On the patient level, ePROs present several benefits: patient awareness of their own health status is increased, and symptoms are more often discussed with providers during follow-up consultations, prompting supportive care measures to be more often put in place [20]. By amplifying the patient's voice, ePROs allow providers to further involve patients in the decision-making process. In oncology patients, early findings indicate a potential overall survival benefit by using ePROs to monitor symptoms followed by remote consultation by healthcare professionals [8, 21]. The following chapter "Utilizing Technology to Manage Symptoms" provides more details of these studies.

Barriers to ePRO implementation include age and computer literacy. Among younger patients, electronic questionnaires collecting PROs are generally preferred to their analogic counterparts for their ease of use [4]. However patients over 70 years old required more assistance with them, which has been attributed to lower computer literacy [4].

Another challenge to ePRO adoption is related to how some of its benefits for patients may not be universal. In oncology, the use of ePROs to remotely monitor symptoms has allowed to decrease the number of emergency admissions [8]. However, this did not apply to patients over 70 years old, who often present multiple comorbidities that require an increased volume of care [22]. Thus, ePRO solutions need to be tailored to the specific characteristics of the population they are intended for, calling for further research before being implemented in routine care.

Challenges to ePRO implementation can also be related to the nature of the data itself, and how it is collected. Legitimate concerns can be raised over the validity and reliability of this data when measures are not standardized. This need has given way to several initiatives: the National Institutes of Health has propelled ePROs with the funding of the Patient-Reported Outcomes Measurement Information System (PROMIS), an initiative to improve the standards for assessing self-reported health status [23]. In oncology, the National Cancer Institute has developed the PRO-CTCAE, a patient-reported outcomes version of the Common Terminology Criteria for Adverse Events (CTCAE) that can be captured electronically [24]. ISPOR has issued recommendations for clinical trials, describing requirements and features for valid ePRO systems [25].

In conclusion, ePRO implementation in routine care can be a challenging endeavor, but rich in opportunities to bring patients and providers closer, with the resulting benefits promising to be greater than the sum of its parts.

Outlook: Real-World Datasets and ePROs in Oncology

As ePROs are now implemented into clinical practice for various patient groups and settings their utility goes beyond clinical care. They are also included in quality and outcome metrics and payer mandates as well as population health and research studies [10].

An example of the potential value of the integration of ePROs in larger datasets is the CANTO study in France. CANTO is a cohort study that led to the creation of a database collecting information in a prospective way on chronic toxicity reported by 20,000 patients treated for localized breast cancer [26]. These data are analyzed by describing chronic toxicity, its incidence, biological characteristics, and clinical manifestations. In addition, this database will allow to evaluate the social impact of chronic toxicity on the quality of life of patients and the economic impact on the cost of cancer treatment. Furthermore, it aims to identify biological markers related to the development of toxicity and develop tests capable of identifying populations at high risk of developing late onset side effects [27].

The integration of ePROs into real-world datasets has the potential to enable the conduct of many studies investigating questions like the CANTO study without needing to set up a study administration for a longitudinal cohort study. We see a rapid development of the real-world datasets for different patient populations. Real-world datasets can be defined as "an umbrella term for different types of healthcare data that are not collected in conventional RCTs. Real world data in the healthcare

Fig. 2 Integration of ePROs in real-world datasets

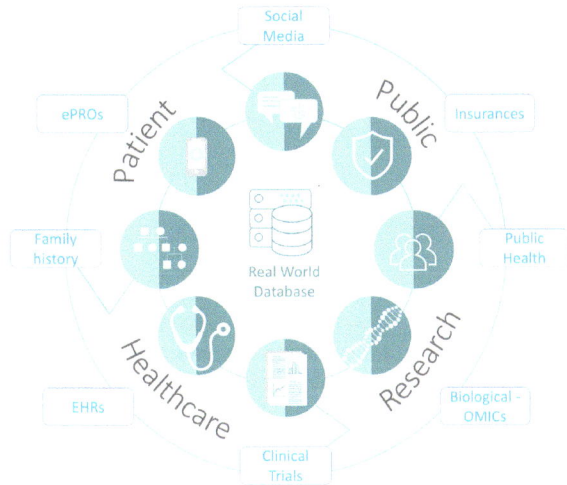

sector come from various sources and include patient data, data from clinicians, hospital data, data from payers, and social data" [28].

The inclusion of ePROs in real-world datasets provides a unique opportunity to perform big data analyses including the patient perspective, investigating its association with a large number of different factors (Fig. 2). The rapid evolution of artificial intelligence might even allow to investigate certain questions in real time, allowing a personalized care approach based on ePROs, clinical, hospital, and social data.

As such, ePROs will continue to gain importance in clinical practice, research, management, and policy making in the future. In this chapter, we highlight the importance of a rigorous and comprehensive development and implementation process to guarantee value of the use of ePROs for patients, clinicians, organizations, and the healthcare system.

References

1. Institute of Medicine (U.S.), Committee on Quality of Health Care in America. Crossing the quality chasm: a new health system for the 21st century. Washington, DC: National Academy Press; 2001. http://public.eblib.com/choice/publicfullrecord.aspx?p=3375215. Accessed 12 Jul 2017.
2. U.S. Food and Drug Administration. Patient-reported outcome measures: use in medical product development to support labeling claims. Washington, DC: U.S. Department of Health and Human Services; 2009. p. 43. (Clinical/Medical).
3. Bingham CO, Noonan VK, Auger C, Feldman DE, Ahmed S, Bartlett SJ. Montreal accord on patient-reported outcomes (PROs) use series – paper 4: patient-reported outcomes can inform clinical decision making in chronic care. J Clin Epidemiol. 2017;89:136–41.

4. Meirte J, Hellemans N, Anthonissen M, Denteneer L, Maertens K, Moortgat P, et al. Benefits and disadvantages of electronic patient-reported outcome measures: systematic review. JMIR Perioper Med. 2020;3(1):e15588.
5. Black N, Burke L, Forrest CB, Ravens Sieberer UH, Ahmed S, Valderas JM, et al. Patient-reported outcomes: pathways to better health, better services, and better societies. Qual Life Res. 2016;25(5):1103–12.
6. Greenhalgh J, Gooding K, Gibbons E, Dalkin S, Wright J, Valderas J, et al. How do patient reported outcome measures (PROMs) support clinician-patient communication and patient care? A realist synthesis. J Patient Rep Outcomes. 2018;2:1. https://doi.org/10.1186/s41687-018-0061-6. Accessed 29 Apr 2020.
7. Howry C, Elash CA, Crescioni M, Eremenco S, O'Donohoe P, Rothrock T. Best practices for avoiding paper backup when implementing electronic approaches to patient-reported outcome data collection in clinical trials. Ther Innov Regul Sci. 2019;53(4):441–5.
8. Basch E, Deal AM, Kris MG, Scher HI, Hudis CA, Sabbatini P, et al. Symptom monitoring with patient-reported outcomes during routine cancer treatment: a randomized controlled trial. J Clin Oncol. 2016;34(6):557–65.
9. Basch E, Deal AM, Dueck AC, Scher HI, Kris MG, Hudis C, et al. Overall survival results of a trial assessing patient-reported outcomes for symptom monitoring during routine cancer treatment. JAMA. 2017;318(2):197.
10. Anastasy C, Barros P, Barry M, Bourek A, Brouwer W, De Maeseneer J, et al. Defining value-based healthcare: report of the expert panel on effective ways of investing in health (EXPH). Luxembourg: Publications Office of the European Union: European Commission; European Union; 2019. p. 94.
11. Penedo FJ, Oswald LB, Kronenfeld JP, Garcia SF, Cella D, Yanez B. The increasing value of eHealth in the delivery of patient-centred cancer care. Lancet Oncol. 2020;21(5):e240–51.
12. Coons SJ, Gwaltney CJ, Hays RD, Lundy JJ, Sloan JA, Revicki DA, et al. Recommendations on evidence needed to support measurement equivalence between electronic and paper-based patient-reported outcome (PRO) measures: ISPOR ePRO Good Research Practices Task Force report. Value Health. 2009;12(4):419–29.
13. Fleischmann M, Vaughan B. The challenges and opportunities of using patient reported outcome measures (PROMs) in clinical practice. Int J Osteopath Med. 2018;28:56–61.
14. WHO Global Observatory for eHealth, World Health Organization. Global diffusion of eHealth: making universal health coverage achievable: report of the third global survey on eHealth. Geneva: WHO; 2016.
15. Lizée T, Basch E, Trémolières P, Voog E, Domont J, Peyraga G, et al. Cost-effectiveness of web-based patient-reported outcome surveillance in patients with lung cancer. J Thorac Oncol. 2019;14(6):1012–20.
16. Byrom B, Tiplady B, editors. ePro: electronic solutions for patient-reported data. Farnham; Burlington, VT: Gower; 2010. 257 p.
17. Coons SJ, Eremenco S, Lundy JJ, O'Donohoe P, O'Gorman H, Malizia W. Capturing patient-reported outcome (PRO) data electronically: the past, present, and promise of ePRO measurement in clinical trials. Patient. 2015;8(4):301–9.
18. European Union. REGULATION (EU) 2016/679 OF THE EUROPEAN PARLIAMENT AND OF THE COUNCIL - of 27 April 2016 - on the protection of natural persons with regard to the processing of personal data and on the free movement of such data, and repealing Directive 95/46/EC (General Data Protection Regulation). 2016. 2016/679, OJ L 119, p 88.
19. PRO-EHR Users' Guide Steering Group, PRO-EHR Users' Guide Working Group, Gensheimer SG, Wu AW, Snyder CF. Oh, the places we'll go: patient-reported outcomes and electronic health records. Patient. 2018;11(6):591–8.
20. Kotronoulas G, Kearney N, Maguire R, Harrow A, Di Domenico D, Croy S, et al. What is the value of the routine use of patient-reported outcome measures toward improvement of patient outcomes, processes of care, and health service outcomes in cancer care? A systematic review of controlled trials. J Clin Oncol. 2014;32(14):1480–501.

21. Denis F, Lethrosne C, Pourel N, Molinier O, Pointreau Y, Domont J, et al. Randomized trial comparing a web-mediated follow-up with routine surveillance in lung cancer patients. J Natl Cancer Inst. 2017;109:9. https://doi.org/10.1093/jnci/djx029/3573360. Accessed 13 Jan 2020.
22. Nipp RD, Horick NK, Deal AM, Rogak LJ, Fuh C, Greer JA, et al. Differential effects of an electronic symptom monitoring intervention based on the age of patients with advanced cancer. Ann Oncol. 2020;31(1):123–30.
23. Cella D, Yount S, Rothrock N, Gershon R, Cook K, Reeve B, et al. The patient-reported outcomes measurement information system (PROMIS): progress of an NIH roadmap cooperative group during its first two years. Med Care. 2007;45(Suppl 1):S3–S11.
24. Basch E, Reeve BB, Mitchell SA, Clauser SB, Minasian LM, Dueck AC, et al. Development of the national cancer institute's patient-reported outcomes version of the common terminology criteria for adverse events (PRO-CTCAE). J Natl Cancer Inst. 2014;106(9):dju244.
25. Zbrozek A, Hebert J, Gogates G, Thorell R, Dell C, Molsen E, et al. Validation of electronic systems to collect patient-reported outcome (PRO) data—recommendations for clinical trial teams: report of the ISPOR ePRO Systems Validation Good Research Practices Task Force. Value Health. 2013;16(4):480–9.
26. Dumas A, Vaz Luis I, Bovagnet T, El Mouhebb M, Di Meglio A, Pinto S, et al. Impact of breast cancer treatment on employment: results of a multicenter prospective cohort study (CANTO). J Clin Oncol. 2020;38(7):734–43.
27. Vaz-Luis I, Cottu P, Mesleard C, Martin AL, Dumas A, Dauchy S, et al. UNICANCER: French prospective cohort study of treatment-related chronic toxicity in women with localised breast cancer (CANTO). ESMO Open. 2019;4(5):e000562.
28. Miani C, Robin E, Horvath V, Manville C, Cave J, Chataway J. Health and healthcare: assessing the real world data policy landscape in Europe. Rand Health Q. 2014;4:15.

Utilizing Technology to Manage Symptoms

Wendy H. Oldenmenger, Corina J. G. van den Hurk, and Doris Howell

Symptom Monitoring and Management in General Healthcare

For many diseases patients use technologies to monitor their symptoms at home and if necessary initiate symptom management. These are called remote symptom monitoring technology (RSMT) and can comprise telemedicine, electronic health (e-health), and mobile health (m-health). Examples include applications to monitor psychotic symptom distress [1], detecting exacerbations of chronic obstructive pulmonary disease [2], recording symptoms of rheumatoid arthritis [3], diabetes mellitus, hemodialysis, or for seasonal allergic rhinoconjunctivitis [4]. The goals of the applications are overall: early detection and intervention, reducing symptoms, and facilitating self-management.

This chapter focuses on cancer-related symptom monitoring and management. In contrast to the above-mentioned diseases, during the often intensive cancer treatment there are many acute symptoms and frequent reporting is indicated. The

W. H. Oldenmenger (✉)
Department of Medical Oncology, Erasmus University Medical Center Cancer Institute, Rotterdam, The Netherlands
e-mail: w.h.oldenmenger@erasmusmc.nl

C. J. G. van den Hurk
Netherlands Comprehensive Cancer Organisation, Utrecht, The Netherlands
e-mail: C.vandenHurk@iknl.nl

D. Howell
Princess Margaret Cancer Centre Research Institute, Toronto, ON, Canada

ELLICSR Health, Wellness and Survivorship Centre, Toronto, ON, Canada

Lawrence Bloomberg Faculty of Nursing and Institute for Health Policy, Management and Evaluation, University of Toronto, Toronto, ON, Canada
e-mail: Doris.Howell@uhn.ca

© Springer Nature Switzerland AG 2020
A. Charalambous (ed.), *Developing and Utilizing Digital Technology in Healthcare for Assessment and Monitoring*,
https://doi.org/10.1007/978-3-030-60697-8_5

subsequent phase of follow-up is comparable for cancer and the other diseases, i.e., the long term and late effects can be monitored less regularly. This chapter mainly addresses acute symptoms that are actively reported by patients.

Symptom Monitoring in Cancer

Online monitoring of patient-reported (PRO) symptoms has proven to be effective in some trials and observational studies among patients with solid tumors [5, 6]. RSMT can add to quality of care and health-related quality of life (HRQoL) of the individual patient. Patients are willing to complete symptom reports and are most compliant if the results are actually used during consultation [7]. If data are fed back to the healthcare provider, there is an immediate overview of what symptoms should be addressed. This is also shown by improved communication about symptoms between patients and healthcare providers [7]. It is also known that the incidence of symptoms is much lower if reported by clinicians, so PRO symptoms give a more comprehensive overview of the patients' experiences at home in between hospital visits [8]. In the phase of follow-up, symptom monitoring showed improved survival among patients with advanced nonprogressive stage IIA to IV lung cancer, because of earlier detection of recurrences [9, 10].

Applications for Symptom Monitoring

Since 2007, several RSMT systems for patients with cancer have been published [6]. We conducted a rapid review using PubMed based on the review of Warrington et al. [6] and found 35 published papers. The search comprised cancer-related online symptom monitoring. Twenty-one papers were from Europe [7, 10–29], 12 from North America [5, 30–40], and two from Asia [41, 42] (Table 1). Fifteen of these studies (43%) were randomized controlled trials; most of the other studies (40%) were feasibility studies. From the initiation of RSMT till today, web-based applications (40%) and mobile devices (26%) or a combination of both were used for symptom monitoring. Since 2016, also four articles about mobile applications have been published. Most articles studied symptom monitoring during the treatment phase of the cancer continuum (91%), mainly during systematic treatment (63%). Only three studies used the symptom monitoring also in follow-up (Table 1).

Content of the Applications

RSMT could comprise several components (Table 1). Only two applications were used solely for assessment/triage of symptoms. Almost all applications (91%) were

Table 1 Overview of symptom monitoring studies

Author	Year	Country	N	Study design	Treatment episode	Target of monitoring	Scoring list	Method	Components Assessment/triage	Monitoring	Education	eConsult	Self-management
Van den Brink	2007	NL	39	nRCT	S	Symptoms	Not specified	Real time at home	–	+	+	+	–
Della Mae	2009	IT	30	FS	ST	CRT	CTCAE	Not real time	–	+	–	–	–
Pfeifer	2015	USA	45	RCT	ST	Symptoms	MSAS	Real time at home	–	+	–	–	–
Kearney	2009	UK	56	RCT	ST	Acute toxicity	Other	Real time and outpatient clinic	–	+	+	–	–
Klasnja	2011	USA	9	FS	ST	Symptoms	Other	Real time at home	–	+	+	–	+
Chan	2013	SG	4	FS	ST	Symptoms	Other	Real time at home	–	+	+	+	–
Nimako	2013	UK	10	FS	ST	CRT	CTCAE	Real time and outpatient clinic	–	+	–	–	–
Ruland	2013	NO	162	RCT	any	Symptoms	MSAS	Real time at home	–	+	+	+	–
Snyder	2013	USA	52	FS	ST	Symptoms	EORTC	Real time and outpatient clinic	–	+	–	+	–

(continued)

Table 1 (continued)

Author	Year	Country	N	Study design	Treatment episode	Target of monitoring	Scoring list	Method	Components Assessment/triage	Monitoring	Education	eConsult	Self-manageme
Berry	2014	USA	374	RCT	any	Symptoms	SDS	Real time at home	–	+	+	–	+
Börösund	2014	NO	111	RCT	ST	Symptoms	MSAS	Real time at home	–	+	+	–	+
Min	2014	KR	30	FS	ST	Sleep	Other	Real time at home	–	+	–	–	–
Weaver	2014	UK	26	FS	ST	Acute toxicity	CTCAE	Real time at home	–	+	–	–	+
Wheelock	2014	USA	59	RCT	FU	Symptoms	MSAS	Real time at home	+	–	+	–	–
Basch	2016	USA	441	RCT	ST	CRT	CTCAE PRO	Real time and outpatient clinic	–	+	–	–	–
Sundberg	2015	SE	9	FS	RT	Symptoms	Not specified	Real time at home	–	+	+	–	+
Egbring	2016	CH	95	RCT	ST	CRT	CTCAE	Not real time	–	+	–	–	–
Foley	2016	IE	13	pRCT	PO	Anxiety	HADS	Not specified	–	–	+	–	–
McGee	2016	UK	18	FS	ST	Symptoms	CSAS	Real time at home	–	+	+	–	+
Peltola	2016	FI	5	FS	RT	Symptoms	CTCAE	Real time and outpatient clinic	–	+	–	+	–

Rasschaert	2016	BE	11	FS	ST	Symptoms	CTCAE	Real time at home	–	+	–	–	–
Steel	2016	USA	144	RCT	any	Symptoms	Not specified	Not real time	–	+	+	–	–
Strasser	2016	CH	145	RCT	ST	Symptoms	ESAS	Outpatient clinic	–	+	–	–	–
Armstrong	2017	CA	32	RCT	S	Pain	PI	Not real time	–	+	–	–	–
Beck	2017	USA	-	DS	ST	Symptoms	Not specified	Real time at home	–	+	+	–	+
Denis	2017	FR	60	RCT	any	Symptoms	Not specified	Real time at home	–	+	–	–	–
Oldenmenger	2017	NL	100	FS	FU	Pain	PI	Real time at home	–	+	+	+	+
Sun	2017	USA	20	FS	S	Symptoms	MDASI	Real time and during admission	–	+	–	–	–
Sundberg	2017	SE	66	nRCT	RT	Symptoms	EORTC	Real time at home	+	+	–	–	–
Coolbrandt	2018	BE	71	CS	ST	CRT	Not specified	Real time at home	–	+	+	–	+
Kolb	2018	USA	121	RCT	ST	Numbness and tingling	Not specified	Real time at home	–	–	–	–	+
Bana	2019	CH	69	DS	ST	CRT	Not specified	Not specified	–	+	+	–	+

(continued)

Table 1 (continued)

Author	Year	Country	N	Study design	Treatment episode	Target of monitoring	Scoring list	Method	Components				
									Assessment/ triage	Monitoring	Education	eConsult	Self-manageme
Van Eenbergen	2020	NL	99	FS	ST	Symptoms	Other	Real time at home	–	+	+	+	+
Greer	2020	USA	91	RCT	ST	Symptoms	MDASI	Real time at home	–	+	+	–	–
Van der Hout	2020	NL	320	RCT	FU	Symptoms	EORTC	Real time at home	–	+	+	–	+

BE Belgium, *CA* Canada, *CH* Switzerland, *FI* Finland, *FR* France, *IE* Ireland, *IT* Italy, *KR* Korea, *NL* Netherlands, *NO* Norway, *SE* Sweden, *SG* Singapore, *UK* United Kingdom, *USA* United States of America, *RCT* randomized controlled trial, *nRCT* non-RCT, *pRCT* pilot RCT, *FS* feasibility study, *DS* development study, *C* cohort study, *ST* systematic therapy, *RT* radiotherapy, *FU* follow-up, *S* surgery, *PO* preoperative, *CRT* common chemo-related toxicity, *EORTC* EORTC QLQC30, *SDS* symptom distress scale, *PI* pain intensity, *CTCAE* common terminology criteria for adverse events, *MSAS* memorial symptom assessment scale, *MDASI* MD Anderson symptom inventory, *HADS* hospital anxiety and depression scale, *CSAS* communication skills attitude scale used to monitor patients' symptoms, 19 applications (54%) included a type of education, and six applications (17%) used an eConsult function to enhance the communication between patients and their healthcare providers. Although most of these symptom monitoring systems were developed to enhance patients' self-management, by means of alert functions and/or advices, this was reported in only a third of the included articles (Table 1).

Using the seven common system features used by Warrington et al. [6], 22/35 of the applications (63%) allowed healthcare professionals to remotely access and monitor patient-reported data; 18/35 of the applications (51%) allowed patients to monitor their symptom reports over time; 17/35 (49%) included a function to send alerts to healthcare providers for severe symptoms; 14/35 of the applications (40%) provided tailored automated patient advice on managing symptoms; 16/35 of the applications (46%) provided general patient information about cancer treatment and side effects; 9/35 of the applications (26%) included a feature for patients to communicate with their healthcare providers; and 4/35 of the applications (11%) included a forum for patients to communicate with one another.

Although all included articles focused on symptom monitoring, the questionnaires were quite heterogeneous. Eight articles described they monitored acute toxicity or common chemo-related toxicity. All other articles reported to monitor "symptoms," or that they monitored a specific symptom like pain or sleep (Table 1). Consequently, different questionnaires were used to monitor these symptoms, among others the Common Toxicity Criteria for Adverse Events (CTCAE) or the Memorial Symptom Assessment Scale (MSAS) (Table 1).

Use and Efficacy of the Applications

Symptom monitoring is primary a nursing intervention. In the articles that described the person who monitors patients' symptoms, this was a nurse (or nurse practitioner) most of the time (74%), followed by a physician (19%) and the clinical team (6%). In two thirds of the included applications an algorithm was used to send alerts to allow healthcare professionals to monitor patients' symptoms or to provide individualized information to the patients. The decisions on what the algorithms were based upon, were not described.

Only 19 articles (54%) reported some kind of efficacy measurements, and most of these studies were randomized controlled trials (Table 2). Twelve of these studies reported on symptoms, and nine of them (75%) found a statistically significant positive effect in favor of the intervention group. The study of Foley et al. described that anxiety and depression scores were significantly lower in the control group where patients did not have access to additional information about these symptoms [21]. Eight studies measured the effect on HRQoL, of which five studies (68%) described a statistically significant positive effect. All five studies measuring the effect on symptom distress reported that patients in the intervention group experienced less

Table 2 Outcomes of symptom monitoring studies

Author	Study design	Quality of life	Symptom distress	Symptoms	Cost-effectiveness	Survival	Self-efficacy
Van den Brink	Non-RCT	+					
Pfeifer	RCT			+			
Kearney	RCT			+			
Ruland	RCT	–	+				–
Berry	RCT		+				
Börösund	RCT		+	+			–
Wheelock	RCT			–			
Basch	RCT	+			+	+	
Egbring	RCT						
Foley	Pilot RCT			!			
Steel	RCT	+		+			
Strasser	RCT			+			
Denis	RCT	+				+	
Oldenmenger	Feasibility			+			
Sundberg	Non-RCT	–		+			
Coolbrandt	Cohort		+	+			+
Kolb	RCT		+	+			
Greer	RCT	–		–			
Van der Hout	RCT	+					–

+ = significant effect; – = nonsignificant effect; ! = significant lower symptoms in control group

symptom distress. Self-efficacy was an endpoint in four studies, of which only one cohort study found a statistically significant effect, while the three RCTs found no effect in these. Two studies reported a statistically significantly longer survival of the patients in the intervention group and only one study measured the cost-effectiveness and reported a statistically significant effect.

All in all, there is huge variation in the content of the RSMT systems, i.e., features as well as number and type of symptoms. Besides, efficacy of the applications is not yet fully proven. The literature showed that symptom monitoring and early intervention against PRO symptoms during active treatment can improve HRQoL and reduce the incidence of severe symptoms [6]. Also, survival might increase because patients remain longer on therapy due to timely symptom management or dose reduction. Patients report a shorter duration of symptoms, and the number of hospital admissions and visits to the emergency department (ED) may decline [5, 8]. Besides advantages for the individual patient, aggregated symptom data can be used as input for shared decision-making and add to deliver value-based healthcare [43] and to write and optimize guidelines for symptom management. The latter can in turn be used for Algorithm-Based Decision Support Systems (AB-DSS).

Algorithm-Based Decision Support Systems

AB-DSS that link patient-reported outcome (PRO) data scores to evidence-based actions are common in written guidelines or "apps" such as the National Comprehensive Cancer Network Guidelines (NCCN), the supportive care guidelines of the Multinational Association of Supportive Care in Cancer (MASCC), and the pan Canadian distress guidelines (Fig. 1) [44]. AB-DSS facilitate clinician decision-making, treatment choices, and reduce variation in evidence-based healthcare [45]. Despite being valued by oncologists and essential for digital ecosystems, their effectiveness in cancer is unclear [46].

AB-DSS for Clinicians

The embedding of AB-DSS within RSMT (mobile, web-based) has been slow to evolve in cancer and as described above wide variation in system features is noted [6]. RSMT may employ simple "if-then" algorithms to compute symptom severity scores from PRO symptom data using established cut-off scores or CTCAE grade levels in "alerting systems." Alerting systems initiate a severe symptom "alert" that is sent to electronic medical records (EMRs) or a separate computer platform for clinicians to view symptom severity graphs over time and handling of alerts. Algorithms may include simple (two paths) AB-DSS alerting on symptom severity

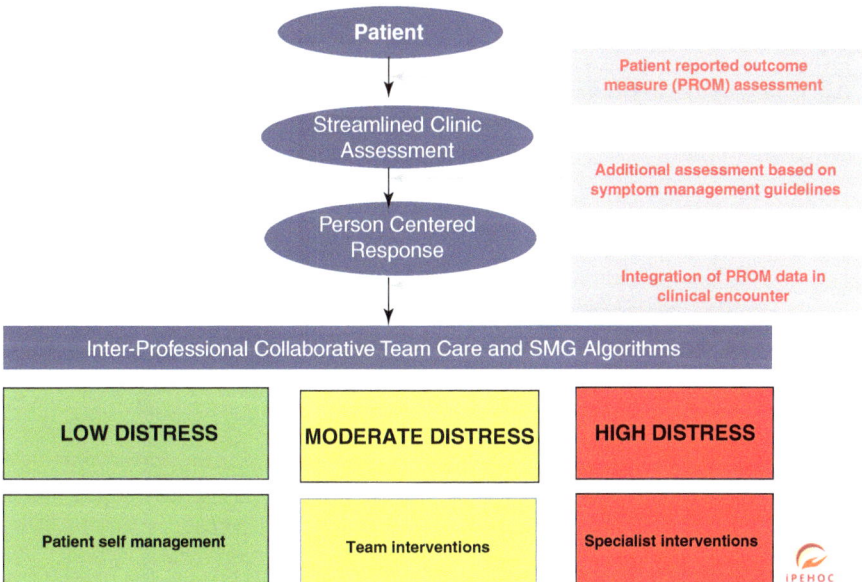

Fig. 1 The Improving Patient Experience and Health Outcome Collaborative (iPEHOC)

and changes in symptoms indicative of worsening taking into consideration previous scores [5, 10]. AB-DSS guidelines are embedded either within these RSMT systems and viewed on the EMR or computer platforms to guide symptom "triage" for handling of alerts. They may as well be disseminated as separate guidance for triage and intensification of "real-time" symptom support by "alert" responders (usually nurses). Some commercial systems (e.g., CAREVIVE@CAREVIVE systems, Inc.) may also generate automated guidance in the form of care plans drawing from evidence-based guidelines such as the NCCN that summarize actions to be taken by patients (self-management actions) and clinicians (treatment plans).

More complex AB-DSS pathways are deployed in some RSMT such as the Advanced Symptom Assessment and Management System (ASyMS) that uses many algorithm-based flow pathways that inform backend computations to derive a range of severity scores (e.g., mild, moderate, or severe). These are in turn combined with other contextual data (i.e., type of chemotherapy agent and/or other symptoms) to create a "risk" score that triggers alerts [13]. In this system two levels of "alerts" are generated to denote the level of urgency for clinician response (i.e., Red = 30 min or Amber = 4 h) (Fig. 2). Other systems, such as the eRapid, also uses complex clinical algorithms to generate "alerts" [47]. Alerting algorithms and threshold scores for alerting were derived through consensus with clinicians. Given the backend computation, these devices are usually designated as medical devices. Similar to eRapid, ASyMS designated triage nurses receive alerts on their phones, view the alert and longitudinal symptom scores on a separate computer platform. It also guides by evidence-based AB-DSS for further telephone triage based on questions for advanced symptom assessment (i.e., extent of interference in functioning due to peripheral neuropathy) and to guide further actions by the patient and/or escalate to urgent care clinics. The research team has further customized the AB-DSS in ASyMS (Can-ASyMS) to align with pan Canadian evidence-informed remote telephone triage guidelines and added contextual data (i.e., symptoms of dehydration) [48].

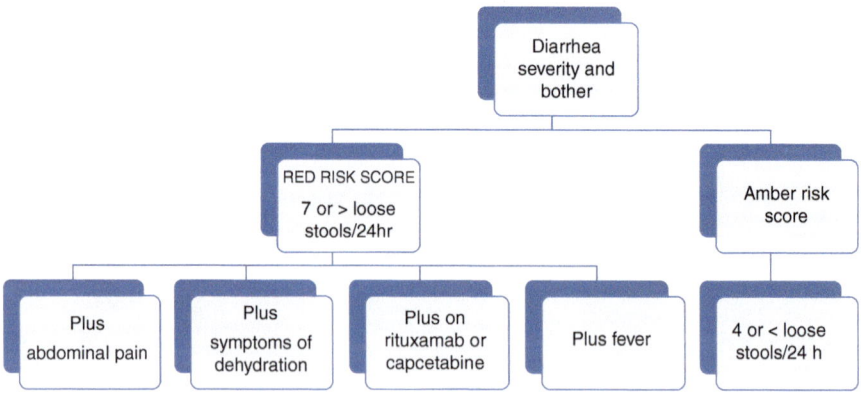

Fig. 2 Algorithm-based flow pathway

As noted in Table 2, there is variability in outcomes for RSMT that may be attributed to differences in the AB-DSS and whether it is embedded or passively disseminated based on an assumption that it will be used by clinicians. Research on RSMT has focused more on outcomes than on underlying mechanisms or care processes that may be causally related to outcome (proximal outcomes), creating a Black Box problem, that makes it difficult to recommend one approach over another [48]. This variation in functionalities and a lack of cost-effectiveness data in studies make it difficult to develop a compelling value-based business case for RSMT integration as a standard of care in cancer systems.

Greater sophistication in the AB-DSS and "alerting systems" within RSMT will need to be considered with the increasing complexity of cancer and treatment (i.e., immunotherapy regimes) and to accommodate multimodal treatment regimes, but concerns have been raised about cognitive overload and the number of decision paths for clinicians when using these systems [49]. Additionally, consensus will need to be reached on both the PRO measures used in RMST (i.e., agnostic or disease or therapy specific) and how these align with other AB-DSS used by clinicians in routine practice. In the future, AB-DSS could be enhanced using computational systems for "alerting systems" that employ artificial intelligence and/or machine learning to inform AB-DSS and risk alerting thresholds in "real time" using big data, but consensus will need to be reached on best practices in computational methods and usability in decision support [50, 51]. Finally, given the real issue of cognitive overload in more complex AB-DSS, cancer programs may need to decide if customization and precision tailoring are embedded fully within the system to address unique patient and/or clinical disease characteristics, and how and what physiological data or omics data can be integrated to inform decision support [52].

Alerting Systems

Greater attention to standardization in AB-DSS and "alerting systems" and the critical threshold scores that indicate risk in cancer is still required and agreement on the problem that these devices are trying to solve including standardization in measurement (i.e., reduce symptom severity and/or ED visits). This is challenging given the diversity of PRO measures used in RSMT (Table 2) and may require cross-walking of scores across different measures (i.e., MSAS vs. PRO-CTCAE) to derive reliable and standard threshold alerts across care systems. In Canada, disease-specific RMST is emerging such as an electronic system for distress screening to be incorporated in patient portals, another mobile system for prostate cancer (NED), and another for chemotherapy (CAN-ASyMS), and for post-surgical monitoring [53]. Overarching digital frameworks require development to guide RSMT deployment in cancer programs and for use of this data in national surveillance.

Consensus also needs to be reached on the right thresholds for "alerting" to ensure differentiation between noise and signal and considering what is reasonable for integration within clinical work flow. Interviews of clinical trial nurses in the Can-ASyMS trial (NCT 03335189) identified that the time to handle an "alert" was on average about 30 min, but could be higher depending on "alert" complexity (i.e., multiple symptom alerts) and patient characteristics. Adherence to alerts as per preset criteria (i.e., 30 min for a red alert) was variable depending on other demands on their time. Alerting systems designed for early identification and intensification of symptom management are only effective if the clinician responds to the alerts. Adherence to alerts was shown to be less than optimal in the Symptom Care@Home trial [37]. Of the 1028 alerts triggered of 457 indicated severe symptoms, there were only 20 provider contacts with the patient. The number of alerts triggered that were not severe is also an example of a "noise vs. signal" problem. RSMT deployed in other diseases have identified "alert fatigue" as a real problem that leads to nonadherence and must be addressed in the design of alerting systems [54].

The increasing complexity of cancer and treatment toxicities (i.e., life threat posed by immunotherapy agents) and the critical alerts that are important and can be sustained in clinical workflow will be crucial for uptake. Functionalities will also need to be developed that avoid continued alerting for symptoms already addressed like in the Dutch SYMPRO trial (NL68440.029.18); otherwise patients may also "hesitate" in reporting severity to avoid needing to wait for a call from the responder if they are already initiating appropriate actions. Healthcare providers need to experience the advantages of RMST first to adapt and invest more time in further implementation and in using the individual results during consultation.

Service Redesign and Implementation

In "real-world" cancer settings, handling alerts and managing patients outside of clinical visits is an "add-on" workload for clinicians who generally do not manage symptoms between clinic visits. RMST deployment will require reconfiguration of clinical workflow and the way team members work together, as existing cancer programs may not be structured to support these in routine cancer care. As noted by Shaw and colleagues, routinized models of care and delivery require disruption and attention to both service design and use of best practices in implementation science [55]. They propose implementation based on a value proposition design approach to guide decisions about tool selection and uptake (i.e., sustainable procurement and PRO), reconfiguration of workflow and team working to respond to PRO data in routine clinical care, and bold organizational leadership and performance governance to sustain uptake. Other issues to be addressed in service design include 24/7 coverage for alert response and designation of responders, longer visit time to handle alerts, access to technology support, educational training, computer literacy of clinicians including interpreting the RSMT output over time, liability and malpractice concerns, privacy protection, regulatory oversight, and reimbursement issues [56]. An equity lens in the design of RSMT and AB-DSS will also be crucial to address population diversity such as age, vulnerability, health, and computer (e-literacy).

AB-DSS to Active Patient Self-Management

Research in other chronic diseases has demonstrated the potential value of RSMT and AB-DSS for improving patient knowledge of disease, fluctuations in symptom patterns over the disease course in self-monitoring, and warning signs of exacerbations [57].

Many RSMTs use AB-DSS to automate delivery of evidence-based, self-care advice to the patients' mobile phone or other web-based platforms tailored to symptom severity levels (i.e., mild or moderate) and adverse events (different advice for pain vs. vomiting) [13, 47]. The structure or content of the self-care advice varies and may replicate written information in educational materials [13] or may be provided as brief coaching messages [37]. It is not clear if self-care advice in RMST conforms to recommendations for action-oriented statements as per the Patient Education Materials Assessment Tool guidelines [58]. While this access to trustworthy self-care information is valuable, it is unclear if this approach translates into better patient activation or self-management behaviors, which are seldom measured (Table 2). If self-care is provided, the application needs to be registered as a medical device.

Passive dissemination of self-care information (actions patients initiate on their own) is overall less effective and differentiated from self-management support for behavior change (SMS) [59]. SMS emphasizes behavior change and patient acquisition of skills inclusive of problem-solving, decision-making, resource utilization, forming a patient-healthcare provider partnership and taking action, and focused on building patient self-efficacy [60]. Comprehensive platforms for SMS are emerging that integrate RSMT and AB-DSS to provide tailored guidance to patients in managing cancer [29].

Future design of RSMT should consider functionality that automates updating of self-care advice and facilitates SMS considering evolving patient capability over the disease course. SMS to address multiple symptoms and emotional consequences of cancer alongside adverse event monitoring will need to be addressed as these interfere with self-management [61]. SMS in RSMT should be deployed as part of "whole system" change towards SMS in cancer care. PRO measures for assessing patient activation, capability, and capacity for self-management should be considered for incorporation in RSMT [62]. Furthermore, nurses responding to alerts will require training in SMS coaching. As noted by Stover and colleagues, self-management advice was provided to 1/3 of the time in response to alerts [63]. Patient/family engagement in deciding on alerting thresholds and self-care advice and SMS may be important as high levels of anxiety were noted for women in response to frequent automated messaging [21].

Finally, social networks and family or informal caregivers play an important role in enabling patient activation in self-management, and consideration will need to be given to features of RSMT that can support their capability. Best practices in design principles and usability to support self-management behaviors [64] and PROs for measurement of these behaviors and self-efficacy will be essential.

Closing Future Considerations

There is a knowledge gap of real-world symptom data during and after cancer treatment. Patient information about symptoms for a particular treatment is currently based on clinician-reported symptoms within trials, which is expected to change if real-time patient-reported symptoms are collected in routine daily care [5]. These data should be validated and forwarded to use in tools, besides SMS also in, e.g., for shared decision-making. Pharmacovigilance centers are also eager to receive this information, as real-world data for medication safety from cancer treatment is scarce. To be able to merge data, researchers and healthcare providers should reach out for more consensus and/or alignment in questionnaires, strive for a common language by using information standards for these questionnaires, and share information, e.g., about algorithms in AB-DSS.

If symptom monitoring applications are used that are linked to other applications and wearables, healthcare providers and/or patients can choose a patient-tailored composition of tools supporting the patient during and following treatment. RSMT, sophisticated AB-DSS, as well as wearables and home blood sample analyses, but also video consulting could prevent patients from unnecessary visits to the hospital. So, there is high potential for symptom monitoring and subsequent management. First steps have been taken, and there is an abundance of possibilities for the future to further improve quality of care and HRQoL.

References

1. Cella M, He Z, Killikelly C, Okruszek L, Lewis S, Wykes T. Blending active and passive digital technology methods to improve symptom monitoring in early psychosis. Early Interv Psychiatry. 2019;13(5):1271–5.
2. Rodriguez Hermosa JL, Fuster Gomila A, Puente Maestu L, Amado Diago CA, Callejas Gonzalez FJ, Malo De Molina Ruiz R, et al. Compliance and utility of a smartphone app for the detection of exacerbations in patients with chronic obstructive pulmonary disease: cohort study. JMIR Mhealth Uhealth. 2020;8(3):e15699.
3. Tam J, Lacaille D, Liu-Ambrose T, Shaw C, Xie H, Backman CL, et al. Effectiveness of an online self-management tool, OPERAS (an on-demand program to EmpoweR Active Self-management), for people with rheumatoid arthritis: a research protocol. Trials. 2019;20(1):712.
4. Di Fraia M, Tripodi S, Arasi S, Dramburg S, Castelli S, Villalta D, et al. Adherence to prescribed E-diary recording by patients with seasonal allergic rhinitis: observational study. J Med Internet Res. 2020;22(3):e16642.
5. Basch E, Deal AM, Kris MG, Scher HI, Hudis CA, Sabbatini P, et al. Symptom monitoring with patient-reported outcomes during routine cancer treatment: a randomized controlled trial. J Clin Oncol. 2016;34(6):557–65.
6. Warrington L, Absolom K, Conner M, Kellar I, Clayton B, Ayres M, et al. Electronic systems for patients to report and manage side effects of cancer treatment: systematic review. J Med Internet Res. 2019;21(1):e10875.
7. van Eenbergen MC, van den Hurk C, Mols F, van de Poll-Franse LV. Usability of an online application for reporting the burden of side effects in cancer patients. Support Care Cancer. 2019;27(9):3411–9.

8. Basch E, Wood WA, Schrag D, Sima CS, Shaw M, Rogak LJ, et al. Feasibility and clinical impact of sharing patient-reported symptom toxicities and performance status with clinical investigators during a phase 2 cancer treatment trial. Clin Trials. 2016;13(3):331–7.
9. Denis F, Basch E, Septans AL, Bennouna J, Urban T, Dueck AC, et al. Two-year survival comparing web-based symptom monitoring vs routine surveillance following treatment for lung cancer. JAMA. 2019;321(3):306–7.
10. Denis F, Lethrosne C, Pourel N, Molinier O, Pointreau Y, Domont J, et al. Randomized trial comparing a web-mediated follow-up with routine surveillance in lung cancer patients. J Natl Cancer Inst. 2017;109(9)
11. van den Brink JL, Moorman PW, de Boer MF, Hop WC, Pruyn JF, Verwoerd CD, et al. Impact on quality of life of a telemedicine system supporting head and neck cancer patients: a controlled trial during the postoperative period at home. J Am Med Inform Assoc. 2007;14(2):198–205.
12. Della Mea V, De Momi I, Aprile G, Puglisi F, Menis J, Casetta A, et al. Feasibility study of a web application for self-report of anticancer treatment toxicities. Stud Health Technol Inform. 2009;150:562–6.
13. Kearney N, McCann L, Norrie J, Taylor L, Gray P, McGee-Lennon M, et al. Evaluation of a mobile phone-based, advanced symptom management system (ASyMS) in the management of chemotherapy-related toxicity. Support Care Cancer. 2009;17(4):437–44.
14. Nimako K, Lu SK, Ayite B, Priest K, Winkley A, Gunapala R, et al. A pilot study of a novel home telemonitoring system for oncology patients receiving chemotherapy. J Telemed Telecare. 2013;19(3):148–52.
15. Ruland CM, Andersen T, Jeneson A, Moore S, Grimsbo GH, Borosund E, et al. Effects of an internet support system to assist cancer patients in reducing symptom distress: a randomized controlled trial. Cancer Nurs. 2013;36(1):6–17.
16. Borosund E, Cvancarova M, Moore SM, Ekstedt M, Ruland CM. Comparing effects in regular practice of e-communication and Web-based self-management support among breast cancer patients: preliminary results from a randomized controlled trial. J Med Internet Res. 2014;16(12):e295.
17. Weaver A, Young AM, Rowntree J, Townsend N, Pearson S, Smith J, et al. Application of mobile phone technology for managing chemotherapy-associated side-effects. Ann Oncol. 2007;18(11):1887–92.
18. Sundberg K, Eklof AL, Blomberg K, Isaksson AK, Wengstrom Y. Feasibility of an interactive ICT-platform for early assessment and management of patient-reported symptoms during radiotherapy for prostate cancer. Eur J Oncol Nurs. 2015;19(5):523–8.
19. Sundberg K, Wengstrom Y, Blomberg K, Halleberg-Nyman M, Frank C, Langius-Eklof A. Early detection and management of symptoms using an interactive smartphone application (Interaktor) during radiotherapy for prostate cancer. Support Care Cancer. 2017;25(7):2195–204.
20. Egbring M, Far E, Roos M, Dietrich M, Brauchbar M, Kullak-Ublick GA, et al. A mobile app to stabilize daily functional activity of breast cancer patients in collaboration with the physician: a randomized controlled clinical trial. J Med Internet Res. 2016;18(9):e238.
21. Foley NM, O'Connell EP, Lehane EA, Livingstone V, Maher B, Kaimkhani S, et al. PATI: patient accessed tailored information: a pilot study to evaluate the effect on preoperative breast cancer patients of information delivered via a mobile application. Breast. 2016;30:54–8.
22. McGee M, Gray P. A handheld chemotherapy symptom management system: results from a preliminary outpatient field trial. Health Informatics J. 2016;11(4):243–58.
23. Peltola MK, Lehikoinen JS, Sippola LT, Saarilahti K, Makitie AA. A novel digital patient-reported outcome platform for head and neck oncology patients-a pilot study. Clin Med Insights Ear Nose Throat. 2016;9:1–6.
24. Rasschaert M, Helsen S, Rolfo C, Van Brussel I, Ravelingien J, Peeters M. Feasibility of an interactive electronic self-report tool for oral cancer therapy in an outpatient setting. Support Care Cancer. 2016;24(8):3567–71.

25. Strasser F, Blum D, von Moos R, Cathomas R, Ribi K, Aebi S, et al. The effect of real-time electronic monitoring of patient-reported symptoms and clinical syndromes in outpatient workflow of medical oncologists: E-MOSAIC, a multicenter cluster-randomized phase III study (SAKK 95/06). Ann Oncol. 2016;27(2):324–32.
26. Oldenmenger WH, Baan MAG, Van der Rijt CCD. Development and feasibility of a web application to monitor patients' cancer-related pain. Support Care Cancer. 2018;26:635–642.
27. Coolbrandt A, Milisen K, Wildiers H, Aertgeerts B, van Achterberg T, Van der Elst E, et al. A nursing intervention aimed at reducing symptom burden during chemotherapy (CHEMO-SUPPORT): a mixed-methods study of the patient experience. Eur J Oncol Nurs. 2018;34:35–41.
28. Bana M, Ribi K, Kropf-Staub S, Zurcher-Florin S, Naf E, Manser T, et al. Implementation of the Symptom Navi (c) Programme for cancer patients in the Swiss outpatient setting: a study protocol for a cluster randomised pilot study (Symptom Navi(c) Pilot Study). BMJ Open. 2019;9(7):e027942.
29. van der Hout A, van Uden-Kraan CF, Holtmaat K, Jansen F, Lissenberg-Witte BI, Nieuwenhuijzen GAP, et al. Role of eHealth application Oncokompas in supporting self-management of symptoms and health-related quality of life in cancer survivors: a randomised, controlled trial. Lancet Oncol. 2020;21(1):80–94.
30. Pfeifer MP, Keeney C, Bumpous J, Schapmire TJ, Studts JL, Myers J, et al. Impact of a tele-health intervention on quality of life and symptom distress in patients with head and neck cancer. J Community Support Oncol. 2015;13(1):14–21.
31. Klasnja P, Hartzler A, Powell C, Pratt W. Supporting cancer patients' unanchored health information management with mobile technology. AMIA Annu Symp Proc. 2011;2011:732–41.
32. Snyder CF, Blackford AL, Wolff AC, Carducci MA, Herman JM, Wu AW, et al. Feasibility and value of PatientViewpoint: a web system for patient-reported outcomes assessment in clinical practice. Psychooncology. 2013;22(4):895–901.
33. Berry DL, Hong F, Halpenny B, Partridge AH, Fann JR, Wolpin S, et al. Electronic self-report assessment for cancer and self-care support: results of a multicenter randomized trial. J Clin Oncol. 2014;32(3):199–205.
34. Wheelock AE, Bock MA, Martin EL, Hwang J, Ernest ML, Rugo HS, et al. SIS.NET: a randomized controlled trial evaluating a web-based system for symptom management after treatment of breast cancer. Cancer. 2015;121(6):893–9.
35. Steel JL, Geller DA, Kim KH, Butterfield LH, Spring M, Grady J, et al. Web-based collaborative care intervention to manage cancer-related symptoms in the palliative care setting. Cancer. 2016;122(8):1270–82.
36. Armstrong KA, Coyte PC, Brown M, Beber B, Semple JL. Effect of home monitoring via mobile app on the number of in-person visits following ambulatory surgery: a randomized clinical trial. JAMA Surg. 2017;152(7):622–7.
37. Beck SL, Eaton LH, Echeverria C, Mooney KH. SymptomCare@Home: developing an integrated symptom monitoring and management system for outpatients receiving chemotherapy. Comput Inform Nurs. 2017;35(10):520–9.
38. Sun V, Dumitra S, Ruel N, Lee B, Melstrom L, Melstrom K, et al. Wireless Monitoring program of patient-centered outcomes and recovery before and after major abdominal cancer surgery. JAMA Surg. 2017;152(9):852–9.
39. Kolb NA, Smith AG, Singleton JR, Beck SL, Howard D, Dittus K, et al. Chemotherapy-related neuropathic symptom management: a randomized trial of an automated symptom-monitoring system paired with nurse practitioner follow-up. Support Care Cancer. 2018;26(5):1607–15.
40. Greer JA, Jacobs JM, Pensak N, Nisotel LE, Fishbein JN, MacDonald JJ, et al. Randomized trial of a smartphone mobile app to improve symptoms and adherence to oral therapy for cancer. J Natl Compr Cancer Netw. 2020;18(2):133–41.

41. Chan MF, Ang E, Duong MC, Chow YL. An online symptom care and management system to monitor and support patients receiving chemotherapy: a pilot study. Int J Nurs Pract. 2013;19(Suppl 1):14–8.

42. Min YH, Lee JW, Shin YW, Jo MW, Sohn G, Lee JH, et al. Daily collection of self-reporting sleep disturbance data via a smartphone app in breast cancer patients receiving chemotherapy: a feasibility study. J Med Internet Res. 2014;16(5):e135.

43. Damman OC, Jani A, de Jong BA, Becker A, Metz MJ, de Bruijne MC, et al. The use of PROMs and shared decision-making in medical encounters with patients: an opportunity to deliver value-based health care to patients. J Eval Clin Pract. 2020;26(2):524–40.

44. Howell D, Keshavarz H, Esplen MJ, Hack T, Hamel M, Howes J, et al. A Pan Canadian practice guideline: screening, assessment and care of psychosocial distress, depression, and anxiety in adults with cancer. Toronto, ON: Canadian Partnership Against Cancer and the Canadian Association of Psychosocial Oncology; 2015.

45. Martínez-Pérez B, de la Torre-Díez I, López-Coronado M, Sainz-de-Abajo B, Robles M, García-Gómez JM. Mobile clinical decision support systems and applications: a literature and commercial review. J Med Syst. 2014;38(1):4.

46. Pawloski PA, Brooks GA, Nielsen ME, Olson-Bullis BA. A systematic review of clinical decision support systems for clinical oncology practice. J Natl Compr Cancer Netw. 2019;17(4):331–8.

47. Holch P, Pini S, Henry AM, Davidson S, Routledge J, Brown J, et al. eRAPID electronic patient self-reporting of adverse-events: patient information and advice: a pilot study protocol in pelvic radiotherapy. Pilot Feasibil Stud. 2018;4:110.

48. Danaher BG, Brendryen H, Seeley JR, Tyler MS, Woolley T. From black box to toolbox: outlining device functionality, engagement activities, and the pervasive information architecture of mHealth interventions. Internet Interv. 2015;2(1):91–101.

49. Walsh S, de Jong EEC, van Timmeren JE, Ibrahim A, Compter I, Peerlings J, et al. Decision support systems in oncology. JCO Clin Cancer Inform. 2019;3:1–9.

50. Naqa IE, Kosorok MR, Jin J, Mierzwa M, Ten Haken RK. Prospects and challenges for clinical decision support in the era of big data. JCO Clin Cancer Inform. 2018;2:1.

51. Kantarjian H, Yu PP. Artificial intelligence, big data, and cancer. JAMA Oncol. 2015;1(5):573–4.

52. Klasnja P, Pratt W. Healthcare in the pocket: mapping the space of mobile-phone health interventions. J Biomed Inform. 2012;45(1):184–98.

53. Avery KNL, Richards HS, Portal A, Reed T, Harding R, Carter R, et al. Developing a real-time electronic symptom monitoring system for patients after discharge following cancer-related surgery. BMC Cancer. 2019;19(1):463.

54. Ancker JS, Edwards A, Nosal S, Hauser D, Mauer E, Kaushal R, et al. Effects of workload, work complexity, and repeated alerts on alert fatigue in a clinical decision support system. BMC Med Inform Decis Mak. 2017;17(1):36.

55. Shaw J, Agarwal P, Desveaux L, Palma DC, Stamenova V, Jamieson T, et al. Beyond "implementation": digital health innovation and service design. NPJ Digit Med. 2018;1:48.

56. Tran C, Dicker AP, Jim HSL. The emerging role of mobile health in oncology. J Target Ther Cancer. 2017;

57. Kim JY, Wineinger NE, Taitel M, Radin JM, Akinbosoye O, Jiang J, et al. Self-monitoring utilization patterns among individuals in an incentivized program for healthy behaviors. J Med Internet Res. 2016;18(11):e292.

58. Shoemaker SJ, Wolf MS, Brach C. The patient educational materials assessment tool (PEMAT) and user's guide. Rockville, MD: Agency for Healthcare Research and Quality, Services UDoHaH; 2013.

59. Grady PA, Gough LL. Self-management: a comprehensive approach to management of chronic conditions. Am J Public Health. 2014;104(8):e25–31.

60. Lorig KR, Holman H. Self-management education: history, definition, outcomes, and mechanisms. Ann Behav Med. 2003;26(1):1–7.

61. Bayliss EA, Ellis JL, Steiner JF. Barriers to self-management and quality-of-life outcomes in seniors with multimorbidities. Ann Fam Med. 2007;5(5):395–402.
62. Hanlon P, Daines L, Campbell C, McKinstry B, Weller D, Pinnock H. Telehealth interventions to support self-management of long-term conditions: a systematic metareview of diabetes, heart failure, asthma, chronic obstructive pulmonary disease, and cancer. J Med Internet Res. 2017;19(5):e172.
63. Stover AM, Tompkins Stricker C, Hammelef K, Henson S, Carr P, Jansen J, et al. Using stakeholder engagement to overcome barriers to implementing patient-reported outcomes (PROs) in cancer care delivery. Approaches from 3 prospective studies. Med Care. 2019;57:S92–S9.
64. Whitehead L, Seaton P. The effectiveness of self-management mobile phone and tablet apps in long-term condition management: a systematic review. J Med Internet Res. 2016;18(5):e97.

Supporting Decision-Making Through Technology

Andreas Charalambous

Introduction

What Is a Clinical Decision-Making in Healthcare?

Decision-making is a key activity in patient–clinician encounters, with decisions as the outcomes of such activity. Clinical decision-making involves the judicious use of evidence, taking into account both clinical expertise and the needs and wishes of individual patients [1].

The term clinical decision-making is not new in healthcare and has received extensive attention in the literature. As a result numerous alternative definitions have been proposed in an effort to describe what the task entails. Variations in the conceptualization of the terms have also been recorded across disciplines. Decision-making can be regarded as the cognitive process resulting in the selection (i.e., which is evidence-based) of a belief or a course of action among several alternative possibilities [2].

Clinical decision-making has often been defined as the process of choosing between alternatives or options [3]. It is a complex process where data are gathered and evaluated, and then a decision, judgment, or intervention is formulated to the best interest of the patient. The complexity lies behind the fact that the healthcare professional must consider numerous, potentially competing factors when making decisions to meet patient and family needs.

Tiffen et al. ([4]: 401) through a multistep development process defined clinical decision-making as a "contextual, continuous, and evolving process, where data are

A. Charalambous (✉)
Nursing Department, Cyprus University of Technology, Limassol, Cyprus

University of Turku, Turku, Finland
e-mail: andreas.charalambous@cut.ac.cy

© Springer Nature Switzerland AG 2020
A. Charalambous (ed.), *Developing and Utilizing Digital Technology in Healthcare for Assessment and Monitoring*,
https://doi.org/10.1007/978-3-030-60697-8_6

gathered, interpreted, and evaluated in order to select an evidence-based choice of action." The definition is supported by a corresponding framework that depicts the clinical decision-making process as an evolving fluid process rather than linear that moves between four steps (data gathering, data interpretation, data evaluation, and decision choice). Based on the underpinnings of this framework, a clinician may begin the process with data gathering and move forward in the process using each step, or the clinician may move in a more iterative manner, depending on attributes of the clinician and the situation [4].

What Is a Clinical Decision Support System?

Clinical decision support systems (CDSSs) or clinical decision support (CDS) are information systems which assist clinical decision-making. Decision support systems are not a novel intervention in healthcare, but rather a mature intervention that has been introduced more than 40 years ago through the seminal work by Shortliffe et al. [5] and others [6–8]. Clinical decision support systems (CDSSs) are platforms that combine multiple clinical data inputs to produce a single output, which can be a diagnosis, clinical advice, or risk stratification that can help clinicians with difficult decision-making [9]. Within healthcare such support systems have been broadly defined by Teich et al. [10] as "providing clinicians with computer-generated clinical knowledge and patient related information which is intelligently filtered and presented at appropriate times to enhance patient care."

Different decision-making tasks may have different features and, therefore, are normally modeled in different forms or presented by different methods and solved by different decision-making techniques. In healthcare decision-making support systems are either knowledge-based or data-driven.

Traditional CDSSs are knowledge-based (KBDSS), where the decisions are from a computerized knowledge base with consideration of the patient characteristics. The underlying technologies for the development of KBDSS can be classified into three categories: technologies for knowledge modeling and representation, technologies for reasoning and inference, and Web-based technologies [11]. These knowledge-based systems serve the purpose of ensuring more accurate decision-making by effectively using timely and appropriate data, information, and knowledge management for convergence industry [12]. Knowledge-based CDSSs rely on relevant knowledge to inform the decision-making process which in turn is based on artificial intelligence and on the application of information and communication technologies. The application of knowledge-based systems in healthcare started in the early 1970s. Since then, KBDSS has been extensively explored to support decision-making in all aspects of healthcare because of the fact that medical conditions are highly diverse, fast changing, and sometimes unpredictable. Preceding studies demonstrate the extensive aspects of where KBDSS has been introduced over time. KBDSS for example has been utilized in clinical pathways as means to standardize medical activities and thereby improve healthcare quality [13] such as through the integration of workflow control into clinical guidelines [14]. There is high value of KBDSS in preventing medical errors when these systems are utilized as clinical risk assessment tools and thus reduce the healthcare service costs caused by patient safety incidents [15].

Data-driven CDSS has been proposed as an alternative approach which uses healthcare big data as the source of information [16]. Data-driven decision-making techniques or called machine-learning-based decision-making techniques are more suitable for an ill-structured decision problem and for decision-making in dynamic and complex situations [17]. These data-driven decision-making systems utilize a range of machine learning applications for analyzing the data by characterizing a decision problem and determining the connections between the problem variables without having explicit knowledge of the physical behavior of the decision model [17]. Xia Jiang et al. [18] developed the Decision Support System for Making Personalized Assessments and Recommendations Concerning Breast Cancer Patients (DPAC), which is a CDSS learned from data that recommends the optimal treatment decisions based on a patient's features. The researchers tested the effectiveness of this data-driven CDSS in a fivefold cross-validation analysis. They compared the probability of being metastasis free in 5 years for patients who made decisions recommended by DPAC to those who did not. They concluded that DPAC is effective at amassing and analyzing data toward treatment recommendations. Nandra et al. [19] utilized Bayesian belief network modeling to develop decision support tools in patients with extremity sarcoma. The aim was to provide a decision support tool that will personalize the short-term survival risk of patients with a diagnosis of bone sarcoma to facilitate complex treatment decisions and align patients' expectations. The researchers generated a Bayesian belief network with five first-degree associates and describe their conditional relationship with survival after the diagnosis of primary bone sarcoma. The factors that predict the outcome of interest, 1-year mortality, in order of relative importance are synchronous metastasis, patient's age, tumor size, histologic grade, and presentation with a pathologic fracture.

The Need for Clinical Decision Support Systems in Healthcare

In order to understand the importance of CDSSs in healthcare one needs to study the clinical context and explicitly the conditions that determined the process of decision-making. The key to successful decision is the timely utilization of all the available data from all the sources. Such clinical data are rapidly expanding and now include (but not limited to) electronic health records (EHRs), disease registries, patient surveys, and information exchanges. It becomes apparent that there is a wealth of quality clinical data (i.e., big data) available per patient that might be overwhelming for clinicians, especially when several complex decisions need to be made in every shift (i.e., during direct patient contact, ward rounds, or multidisciplinary meetings) and in a very short time. Although the combination of big data and digitalization provides a solution to the problem, it does not ensure better or safer patient care [20, 21]. This is where the value of CDSS tools lies, by incorporating big data and digitalization in a single solution that can provide high-quality clinical decision support. As discussed earlier, decision-making in the healthcare context is a highly complex and demanding process that can be further complicated by the fact that healthcare providers often do not know that certain patient data are available in the EHR, do not always know how to access the data, do not have the time to search for the data, or are not fully informed on the most current medical insights [22, 23].

The aim of CDSSs is to strengthen the decision-making process by incorporating a wealth of evidence and knowledge contrary to current decisions that are determined by the experience and knowledge of the clinician. A number of CDSSs implement some kind of artificial intelligence named machine learning that allows computer to learn from past experiences and/or detect figures from clinical data. This property of the CDSS allows the clinician to have an ongoing monitoring of the patient's status instead of fragmented snapshots taken during clinic visits or admissions. Therefore, machine learning can enable the detection of subtle irregularities in the patient's condition that are difficult to be captured by clinicians within the scope of the profession.

Utilizing Clinical Decision Support Systems in Healthcare

The complexity of the clinical decision-making landscape in healthcare has facilitated the rise of an increased number of applications in medical and nursing science as well as either disciplines and professions, both within the hospital and in ambulatory care settings. The most common types of CDSS in healthcare include drug-interaction checking, preventive care reminders, and automatic adverse-event detection. Furthermore, the CDSS can check for patient drug allergies, compare drug and laboratory values, suggest drug alternatives, block duplicate orders, suggest drug doses, routes, and frequencies, and provide recommendations.

As the complexity of clinical practice continues to grow, so are the challenges posed by clinical decision-making. For example, along with the growth of standardized patient pathways, a key issue concerns the decision to initiate a pathway combining both administrative and clinical prescriptions for a particular patient [24]. Accordingly, the use of patient pathways addresses a need to identify patients who will benefit from a particular pathway, due to limited resources within the healthcare service in general [25]. In an acute care environment, nurses are often providing care to several patients, limiting therefore the time for efficient decision-making or increasing the stress of making appropriate decisions in life-threatening scenarios [26]. De Bock et al. [27] showed that the organization and structure of the many practices in a hospital are crucial in decision-making processes. These practices result in many occasions in practitioners to shift in their decision-making from an analytic to a complex approach.

The decision-making support tools are designed to support clinicians across the disease trajectory from preventive care through diagnosis, planning, and treatment to monitoring and follow-up [28]. Although these decision support systems have numerous implications, they have been widely applied in data analysis, on-demand access to practice guidelines, active symptom management, to avoid medical errors to mention a few.

An area in clinical practice where such decision support systems have been utilized both by medical doctors and nurses is the accident and emergency departments (EDs) where critical decisions need to be made in a relatively short period of time. Within this context, Triage is a complex decision-making process, and several triage scales have been designed as decision support systems to guide the triage nurse to a correct decision [29]. The aim of triage scales is to minimize the waiting time of patients according to the severity of their medical condition, in order to treat the most intense symptoms as quickly as possible and to reduce the negative impact on the prognosis of a prolonged delay before treatment. An example of such a triage scale that it is based on a DSS is the Rapid Emergency Triage and Treatment System (M(R)ETTS) which is widely used at the EDs [30]. Nurses recognize patient deterioration (which requires situational awareness) and determine which patient conditions have clinical guidelines that apply, which nursing interventions are appropriate, and what are ways to promote patient centeredness of medical interventions [31]. The value of such support systems is essential in chronic diseases that often involve unpredictable disease developments that require complex disease management strategies [32]. Chronic obstructive pulmonary disease (COPD) is such a chronic condition that requires advanced management. The challenges presented by COPD are demonstrated by Velickovski et al. [33] who developed a DSS that offers a suite of services for the early detection and assessment of COPD. In order to provide comprehensive and efficient management of COPD, researchers had to develop a suite of decision support web services for (1) COPD early detection and diagnosis, (2) spirometry quality control support, and (3) patient stratification in a secured environment online.

Challenges for Clinical Decision Support Systems

Numerous computerized decision support systems (CDSSs) and other aids have been developed to assist patient management across diseases and clinical contexts. However, systematic reviews show that such support systems are not consistently effective in demonstrating outcome improvements or highly significant results (e.g., at improving decisions) [34]. In an early systematic review by Garg et al. [28] of controlled trials of DSSs, the findings showed that one third of the studies were not effective at narrowing knowledge gaps, improving decisions, clinical practice, or patient outcomes. In a subsequent systematic review, Jaspers et al. [35] synthesized the literature on CDSS's impact on healthcare practitioner performance and patient outcomes. Evidence that CDSS significantly impacted practitioner performance was found in 52 out of 91 unique studies of the 16 SRs examining this effect (57%). Only 25 out of 82 unique studies of the 16 SRs reported evidence that CDSS positively impacted patient outcomes (30%). Bright et al. [36] undertook a systematic review of randomized trials to evaluate the effect of CDSSs on clinical outcomes, healthcare processes, workload and efficiency, patient satisfaction, cost, and provider use and implementation. Clinical decision support had a favorable effect on prescribing treatments, facilitating preventive care services, and ordering clinical studies across diverse venues and systems. Evidence demonstrating positive effects of CDSSs on clinical and economic outcomes remains surprisingly sparse and safe conclusions cannot be drawn. A systematic review and meta-analysis was conducted to provide insight into the effects of computerized decision support systems (CDSS) on cardiovascular risk factor levels and identify characteristics of CDSS related to improved care [37]. The authors concluded that although a considerable number of CDSS for cardiovascular risk management (CVRM) were developed, a clear clinical benefit is absent.

A systematic review by Melton [38] sought to assess the applications and implications of current medical informatics-based decision support systems related to medication prescribing and use. Medical informatics-based decision support has potential to positively impact not only patient safety and outcomes but also workflow efficiency. However, the results showed that in a number of studies, increased number of errors or delays in care were recorded as a result of decision support. This finding was partially attributed to poor design or usability and may be avoided with further testing and refinement of the interfaces themselves.

These systematic reviews revealed several challenges for the wide utilization of CDSS in clinical practice. These challenges can be divided into three levels including the knowledge/data base that forms the CDSS, the methodological challenges, and finally the ethical concerns raised. CDSSs rely heavily on the quality and completeness of patient-related data (i.e., real world data) in order to inform timely and effective decision-making. Therefore, the widespread access to biomedical data, the transfer of big data knowledge into point-of-care systems, and the exploitation of patient-reported outcome measures in real-time care through patient engagement are only some of the issues that pose challenges to the development and effective utilization of CDSS. Explicitly for patient involvement in the CDSS process, studies showed that they increase the effects of the support systems [37]. These issues can also interact with other factors resulting in a negative impact on the low clinical utilization of CDSS. Such factors might include the poor design of the human interface, imposing changes and failing to fit naturally into the routine workflow, and resistance or computer illiteracy of some healthcare workers to report a few [39]. As revealed by the above systematic reviews and others, there are several methodological challenges that have been reported as barriers to the development and widespread utilization of CDSS. Issues for example on how to optimize data calibration with discrimination in predictive learning models, or how to ensure accurate probability estimations for risk assessment, diagnosis, therapeutic intervention, and prognosis need to be considered and addressed. Another methodological challenge to be considered in this context is the fact that CDSSs focus primarily on guideline adherence management measured by change in pharmacological treatment and risk factor profiles without registering meta-information on the decisions. This creates a knowledge gap that affects the uptake of the CDSS as there are no information on the way that the CDSS affected counseling by the physician and the shared decision-making process. There are several areas of ethical concern that have arisen in regard to CDSS such as the effect of the system on the standard of care. This refers to whether the system improves patient care and helps providers fulfill the responsibilities placed upon them by society [40]. Within the context of CDSS, the provider is the ultimate decision-maker; however ethical concerns can be raised if the provider relies on decision support recommendations that prove incorrect [41] or the system is not used by appropriately trained personnel for the purpose it was designed for [42]. Other potential sources of ethical concerns include the extent an algorithm can influence decisions on probabilistically determined critical conditions or what hierarchy of evidence can guide clinical decision-making at reduced risk of bias and whether expensive therapies be considered when facing marginal survival chances [34].

How Would Clinical Decision Support Tools Be Designed?

CDSSs in principle enable the clinician to integrate evidence and patient information (i.e., from multiple resources) into tailored strategies for daily practice and increase guideline adherence. Explicitly, preceding studies showed that CDSS can be beneficial in providing guidance with clinical practice problems and improve the overall efficiency and quality of healthcare delivery systems [43, 44]. Early systematic reviews [45] as well as subsequent ones [36] provide evidence on the value of CDSSs in increasing the use of preventive care in hospitalized patients, facilitate communication between providers and patients, and enable faster and more accurate access to medical record data. However, as discussed above, the introduction of CDSS into a complex environment such as the one in healthcare needs the consideration of many factors to enable such systems to operate effectively and have a meaningful clinical impact. The fact that the clinical contexts where the CDSS is intended to be used (e.g., oncology, cardiology) can differ significantly for example in relation to the amount of available information (e.g., in the form of guidelines) and level of usability and integration in clinical practice makes it difficult to suggest a universal "Golden Standard" for the development of such CDSS. Therefore what is attempted in this section is to identify and discuss those critical design criteria for CDSS that can make their utilization efficient, effective, and safe.

In a narrative review of design and functional requirements for clinical decision support, Miller et al. [46] identified design recommendations for CDSS to support the efficient, effective, and timely delivery of high-quality care. The authors classified these recommendation in the following three categories: interface features, information features, and interaction features. Interface features include the presentation, placement, and positioning and provision of multiple presentation layers.

These subcategories represent issues related to the simplicity and visibility of the information provided as well as usability easiness of the interface. Information features can be summarized in information that are presented in a consistent way (i.e., consistent way recommendations are presented), which are relevant to those who can act on the information and demonstrate clarity by being presented as clean and concise. In a synthesis of systematic reviews, it was demonstrated that the efficacy of CDSS can be improved when the specificity and sensitivity levels of their advice increase [35]. The information provided to clinicians not only needs to be concise and specific but also needs to take into consideration the level of priority (e.g., life-threatening alert). Preceding studies have found up to 95% of CDSS alerts are inconsequential, and often clinicians disagree with or distrust alerts [42]. There is a risk that if physicians are presented with excessive/unimportant alerts, they can suffer from alert fatigue that can be the source of errors [47].

In the category of interface features several elements have been identified such as the ability of CDSS to timely deliver recommendations and use in a way that complex data can be rapidly accessible and easily understood within a provider's workflow (i.e., minimizing user's cognitive load). CDSS should have the ability to send information back to the user about what action has been done and what result was accomplished (feature of feedback) automatically as part of clinician workflow (i.e., CDSS is provided at the point of care or order). Kawamoto et al. [48] found that the most effective CDS has four components: it is designed in line with workflow ($p < 0.001$), offers recommendations with assessments ($p = 0.019$), provides guidance at the time and location when decisions are made ($p = 0.026$), and is computer based ($p = 0.029$). The authors concluded that of systems that had all four components, 94% showed benefit.

Clinical contexts are complex and dynamic and therefore are characterized by constant and sudden change of circumstances. CDSSs need to take this into consideration, and therefore be flexible and adaptable, able to explore multiple assumptions, and incorporate new information as circumstances change [46]. Therefore, the information that CDSSs provide needs to reflect the decision-making process and the intellectual effort of clinicians in a contextually relevant way. CDSS should make dynamic predictions, allowing interactions with clinicians and taking into consideration the longitudinal nature of health and disease [49].

Conclusion

Clinicians are involved in decision-making tasks throughout their shifts in mostly every managing action in relation to patients' conditions. Clinical decision support systems have changed (i.e., where such systems have been introduced) the way that clinical decision-making is undertaken in healthcare. These systems have been developed specifically to provide clinicians with relevant knowledge, intelligently filtered or presented at appropriate times, to enhance health and healthcare, and positive outcomes have been recorded in terms of patient safety, quality, and efficient care. CDSSs are especially important when the situation is rapidly changing, and anticipation and determination of future situations/conditions are hardly possible. The recognition of CDSS as an effective pathway to minimize errors in clinical practice has gained momentum, and its utilization in practice continues to expand. As institutions work toward Meaningful Use, medical informatics-based decision support will continue to grow in importance as more studies are produced, which show these systems benefit patients and providers.

The high adoption and effective use of CDSS depend largely on the quality of the system design. Preceding studies have documented that effective decision support must be carefully designed to fit within clinical workflows (e.g., deployed across diverse settings), and these workflows depend on how clinicians and patients approach decision-making and how they choose to interact. From the user's perspective it is essential that the information delivered by the CDSS is directed at the appropriate members of the care team in minimally disruptive and explicit way (i.e., right information to clinicians in the correct format and at the right time). Future research should focus on ensuring the accuracy and effectiveness of systems to maximize patient safety and minimize alert fatigue.

The evolution of CDSSs has progressed expediently in the field of healthcare, and it is now utilized across the disease continuum. However, there are areas where CDSSs need to be expanded even more to be in accordance with the complexities of clinical disease management. An area that requires further development is the compatibility of current or newly designed CDSSs to accommodate multiple comorbid conditions simultaneously. The management of multimorbid patients is complex because the number of risk factors increases with the number of clinical conditions [50]. Multimorbid conditions affect each other and are closely associated with mortality, severe disability, care variations, increased health resource use, and costs [51]. With the prevalence of multimorbidity on the rise, it becomes essential to develop CDSSs that effectively incorporate the clinical needs dictated by the multiple diseases.

Clinical decision support systems have proven to be effective in improving many aspects of decision-making in the field of healthcare. In a highly complex clinical environment where the management of patients is becoming increasingly challenging, CDSS tools can be a valuable pathway to support patients, families as well as clinicians in the decision-making process.

References

1. Bate L, Hutchinson A, Underhill J, Maskrey N. How clinical decisions are made. Br J Clin Pharmacol. 2012;74(4):614–20. https://doi.org/10.1111/j.1365-2125.2012.04366.x.
2. Ofstad EH, Frich JC, Schei E, Frankel RM, Gulbrandsen P. What is a medical decision? A taxonomy based on physician statements in hospital encounters: a qualitative study. BMJ Open. 2016;6(2):e010098. https://doi.org/10.1136/bmjopen-2015-010098.

3. Thompson C, Stapley S. Do educational interventions improve nurses' clinical decision making and judgement? A systematic review. Int J Nurs Stud. 2011;48:881–93. https://doi.org/10.1016/j.ijnurstu.2010.12.005.
4. Tiffen J, Corbridge SJ, Slimmer L. Enhancing clinical decision making: development of a contiguous definition and conceptual framework. J Prof Nurs. 2014;30(5):399–405. https://doi.org/10.1016/j.profnurs.2014.01.006.
5. Shortliffe EH, Davis R, Axline SG, et al. Computer-based consultations in clinical therapeutics: explanation and rule acquisition capabilities of the MYCIN system. Comput Biomed Res. 1975;8(4):303–20.
6. Lamott K. Using computers in planning and programming. Hospitals. 1967;41:127.
7. Lindberg D. Collection, evaluation, and transmission of hospital laboratory data. Methods Inf Med. 1967;6:97.
8. Long JM, Flanigan WJ, Hara M, Levy GC. Planning and managing new and complex medical and surgical procedures. JAMA. 1966;196:161.
9. Hagiwara MA, Sjöqvist BA, Lundberg L, Suserud B-O, Henricson M, Jonsson A. Decision support system in prehospital care: a randomized controlled simulation study. Am J Emerg Med. 2013;31(1):145–53. https://doi.org/10.1016/j.ajem.2012.06.030.
10. Teich JM, Osheroff JA, Pifer EA, Sittig DF, Jenders RA. Clinical decision support in electronic prescribing: recommendations and an action plan. J Am Med Inform Assoc. 2005;12(4): 365–76.
11. Zaraté P, Liu S. A new trend for knowledge-based decision support systems design. Int J Inf Decis Sci. 2016;8(3):305–24.
12. Chung K, Boutaba R, Hariri S. Knowledge based decision support system. Inf Technol Manag. 2016;17:1–3. https://doi.org/10.1007/s10799-015-0251-3.
13. Yang H, Li W, Liu K, Zhang J. Knowledge-based clinical pathway for medical quality improvement. Inf Syst Front. 2011;14(1):105–17.
14. Lee J, Jang J, Shim B, Kim ST, Kim HY, Song S, Kim J, Cho I, Kim YA. Workflow based clinical decision support system through integration of clinical workflow and knowledge processing. Int J Innov Comput Inf Contr. 2012;8(7):5251–64.
15. Kong G, Xu DL, Body R, Yang JB, Mackway-Jones K, Carley S. A belief rule-based decision support systems for clinical risk assessment. Eur J Oper Res. 2012;219:564–73.
16. Dagliati A, Tibollo V, Sacchi L, Malovini A, Limongelli I, Gabetta M, Napolitano C, Mazzanti A, De Cata P, Chiovato L, Priori S, Bellazzi R. Big data as a driver for clinical decision support systems: a learning health systems perspective. Front Digit Humanit. 2018;5:8. https://doi.org/10.3389/fdigh.2018.00008.
17. Lu J, Liu A, Song Y, et al. Data-driven decision support under concept drift in streamed big data. Complex Intell Syst. 2020;6:157–63. https://doi.org/10.1007/s40747-019-00124-4.
18. Jiang X, Wells A, Brufsky A, Neapolitan R. A clinical decision support system learned from data to personalize treatment recommendations towards preventing breast cancer metastasis. PLoS One. 2019;14(3):e0213292. https://doi.org/10.1371/journal.pone.0213292.
19. Nandra R, Parry M, Forsberg J, Grimer R. Can a Bayesian belief network be used to estimate 1-year survival in patients with bone sarcomas. Clin Orthop Relat Res. 2017;475(6):1681–9. https://doi.org/10.1007/s11999-017-5346-1.
20. Magrabi F, Ammenwerth E, Hypponen H, de Keizer N, Nykanen P, Rigby M, et al. Improving evaluation to address the unintended consequences of health information technology: a position paper from the Working Group on Technology Assessment & Quality Development. Yearb Med Inform. 2016;1:61–9.
21. Lehmann CU, Seroussi B, Jaulent MC. Troubled waters: navigating unintended consequences of health information technology. Yearb Med Inform. 2016;1:5–6.
22. Mamlin BW, Tierney WM. The promise of information and communication technology in healthcare: extracting value from the chaos. Am J Med Sci. 2016;351(1):59–68.
23. Wasylewicz ATM, Scheepers-Hoeks AMJW. Clinical decision support systems. In: Kubben P, Dumontier M, Dekker A, editors. Fundamentals of clinical data science. Cham: Springer; 2019.

24. Fraccaro P, Casteleiro MA, Ainsworth J, Buchan I. Adoption of clinical decision support in multimorbidity: a systematic review. JMIR Med Inform. 2015;3:1. https://doi.org/10.2196/medinform.3503.
25. Møller NH, Bjørn P. Layers in sorting practices: sorting out patients with potential cancer. Comput Support Cooperat Work. 2011;20(3):123–53. https://doi.org/10.1007/s10606-011-9133-3.
26. Nibbelink CW, Brewer BB. Decision-making in nursing practice: an integrative literature review. J Clin Nurs. 2018;27(5–6):917–28. https://doi.org/10.1111/jocn.14151.
27. de Bock BA, Willems DL, Weinstein HC. Complexity perspectives on clinical decision making in an intensive care unit. J Eval Clin Pract. 2018;24:308–13. https://doi.org/10.1111/jep.12794.
28. Garg AX, Adhikari NKJ, McDonald H, Rosas-Arellano MP, Devereaux PJ, Beyene J, et al. Effects of computerized clinical decision support systems on practitioner performance and patient outcomes: a systematic review. JAMA. 2005;293(10):1223–38.
29. Kihlgren A, Svensson F, Lövbrand C, et al. A decision support system (DSS) for municipal nurses encountering health deterioration among older people. BMC Nurs. 2016;15:63. https://doi.org/10.1186/s12912-016-0184-0.
30. Vicente V. The use of a prehospital decision system in the emergency medical service – the acute emergency chain for geriatric patients. Thesis. Stockholm: Karolinska Institutet; 2013. ISBN 978-91-7549-021-2.
31. Lopez KD, Gephart SM, Raszewski R, Sousa V, Shehorn LE, Abraham I. Integrative review of clinical decision support for registered nurses in acute care settings. J Am Med Inform Assoc. 2017;24(2):441–50. https://doi.org/10.1093/jamia/ocw084.
32. Oudshoorn N. Telecare technologies and the transformation of health care. Basingstoke: Palgrave McMillian; 2016.
33. Velickovski F, Ceccaroni L, Roca J, et al. Clinical Decision Support Systems (CDSS) for preventive management of COPD patients. J Transl Med. 2014;12(Suppl 2):S9. https://doi.org/10.1186/1479-5876-12-S2-S9.
34. Capobianco E. Data-driven clinical decision processes: it's time. J Transl Med. 2019;17(1):44. https://doi.org/10.1186/s12967-019-1795-5.
35. Jaspers MW, Smeulers M, Vermeulen H, Peute LW. Effects of clinical decision-support systems on practitioner performance and patient outcomes: a synthesis of high-quality systematic review findings. J Am Med Inform Assoc. 2011;18(3):327–34. https://doi.org/10.1136/amiajnl-2011-000094.
36. Bright TJ, Wong A, Dhurjati R, Bristow E, Bastian L, Coeytaux RR, Samsa G, Hasselblad V, Williams JW, Musty MD, Wing L, Kendrick AS, Sanders GD, Lobach D. Effect of clinical decision-support systems: a systematic review. Ann Intern Med. 2012;157(1):29–43. https://doi.org/10.7326/0003-4819-157-1-201207030-0045.
37. Groenhof TKJ, Asselbergs FW, Groenwold RHH, et al. The effect of computerized decision support systems on cardiovascular risk factors: a systematic review and meta-analysis. BMC Med Inform Decis Mak. 2019;19:108. https://doi.org/10.1186/s12911-019-0824-x.
38. Melton BL. Systematic review of medical informatics-supported medication decision making. Biomed Inform Insights. 2017;9:1178222617697975. https://doi.org/10.1177/1178222617697975.
39. Blake JN, Kerr DV, Gammack GJ. Streamlining patient consultations for sleep disorders with a knowledge-based CDSS. Inf Syst. 2016;56:109–19.
40. Goodman KW. Ethical and legal issues in decision support. In: Berner ES, editor. Clinical decision support systems. Health informatics. New York, NY: Springer; 2007.
41. Phillips W. Ethical controversies about proper health informatics practices. Mo Med. 2015;112(1):53–7.
42. Sutton RT, Pincock D, Baumgart DC, Sadowski DC, Fedorak RN, Kroeker KI. An overview of clinical decision support systems: benefits, risks, and strategies for success. NPJ Digit Med. 2020;3:17. https://doi.org/10.1038/s41746-020-0221-y.

43. Moja L, Kwag KH, Lytras T, et al. Effectiveness of computerized decision support systems linked to electronic health records: a systematic review and meta-analysis. Am J Public Health. 2014;104(12):e12–22. https://doi.org/10.2105/AJPH.2014.302164.
44. Roshanov PS, Fernandes N, Wilczynski JM, et al. Features of effective computerised clinical decision support systems: meta-regression of 162 randomised trials. BMJ. 2013;346:f657.
45. Kaushal R, Shojania KG, Bates DW. Effects of computerized physician order entry and clinical decision support systems on medication safety: a systematic review. Arch Intern Med. 2003;163(12):1409–16.
46. Miller K, Mosby D, Capan M, et al. Interface, information, interaction: a narrative review of design and functional requirements for clinical decision support. J Am Med Inform Assoc. 2018;25(5):585–92. https://doi.org/10.1093/jamia/ocx118.
47. Khalifa M, Zabani I. Improving utilization of clinical decision support systems by reducing alert fatigue: strategies and recommendations. Stud Health Technol Inform. 2016;226:51–4.
48. Kawamoto K, Houlihan CA, Balas EA, Lobach DF. Improving clinical practice using clinical decision support systems: a systematic review of trials to identify features critical to success. BMJ. 2005;330(7494):765.
49. Zikos D, DeLellis N. CDSS-RM: a clinical decision support system reference model. BMC Med Res Methodol. 2018;18:137. https://doi.org/10.1186/s12874-018-0587-6.
50. Bilici E, Despotou G, Arvanitis TN. The use of computer-interpretable clinical guidelines to manage care complexities of patients with multimorbid conditions: a review. Digit Health. 2018;4:2055207618804927.
51. Vassilaki M, Aakre JA, Cha RH. Multimorbidity and risk of mild cognitive impairment. J Am Geriatr Soc. 2015;63(9):1783–90.

Virtual Reality and Augmeneted Reality for Managing Symptoms

Andreas Charalambous and Androniki Ioannou

Introduction

Nowadays, Virtual Reality (VR) and Augmented Reality (AR) are technological solutions that their popularity is ever increasing. As the underlying technology and software are evolving, VR and AR have been commonly used in many fields, such as health services and hospitality, education, tourism, cultural, military, construction, design, engineering, gaming, and entertainment [1].

In VR, the user is able to immerse and interact with the system technology but all the images displayed are virtual. VR is the virtual construction of an artificial world. The key element of VR is the high level of user's immersion over the virtual environment, as well as the interaction of the user with the environment in a realistic way [2]. In another interesting way, people have described the experience as being a "spiritual journey." On the other hand, Augmented Reality is a view of a real-world physical environment or object seen by a mobile phone, tablet, or AR glasses, whose elements are augmented by computer-generated input. AR presents a semi-true and false image, which is the combination of real and virtual; some people commonly describe it as the "third eye" [3].

Milgram, Takemura, Utsumi, and Kishino place AR and VR in a continuum line. AR is in between reality (real environment) and virtuality (virtual environment) on

A. Charalambous (✉)
Nursing Department, Cyprus University of Technology, Limassol, Cyprus

University of Turku, Turku, Finland
e-mail: andreas.charalambous@cut.ac.cy

A. Ioannou
Cyprus University of Technology, Limassol, Cyprus

© Springer Nature Switzerland AG 2020
A. Charalambous (ed.), *Developing and Utilizing Digital Technology in Healthcare for Assessment and Monitoring*,
https://doi.org/10.1007/978-3-030-60697-8_7

the reality-virtuality continuum. This is a continuous scale ranging between reality, where everything is physical, and virtual reality, where a complete virtual environment is created by a computer. Mixed reality is located between them and includes AR and augmented virtuality (AV) [4, 5].

Media reported 2016 as the year that VR and AR being popularized. Many video platforms such as YouTube and Vimeo have started to support VR applications and VR video watching followed by an increasing number of museums offering a VR navigation experience [6].

The healthcare market of VR and AR will reach 2.54 billion U.S. dollars by 2020, mainly including surgical applications, medical rehabilitation, medical consultation, medical diagnosis, and medical education and training [7]. These technologies can be utilized in many settings to assist in health behavior change interventions, optimize care, and improve health outcomes of individuals across all care settings [8].

Virtual Reality

What Is VR?

The term virtual reality (VR) was used for the first time in 1989 by Jaron Lamier. The most popular definition of VR refers to a particular technological system, which includes a computer capable of providing interactive three-dimensional (3D) visualization, a controller for interaction with the animations, a position tracker, and a head-mounted display (HMD) to deliver the visual output. The trackers monitor the position and orientation of the user in space and provide the information to the computer that updates in real time the images for display [9–11].

In their reviews about the use of VR in healthcare, Rubino et al. [12], McCloy and Stone [13], and Székely and Satava [14] share this vision: "VR is a collection of technologies that allow people to interact efficiently with 3D computerized databases in real time using their natural senses and skills." Rizzo and Wiederhold [15] defined VR as "an advanced interface that allows the user to 'interact' with and become 'immersed' within a computer generated environment."

VR Technology

VR is immersive and interactive, engaging several senses simultaneously. This technology allows an individual to hear and feel stimuli that correspond with a visual image. VR does not require practice prior to use in the clinical setting. The headset provides an enclosed visual environment and supplies the person with distracting images that can be a reproduction of an actual environment or a manufactured fictional one [16–18].

VR technology has advanced to such an extent that it has become well established in immersive and interactive environments: immersive, because users have the sense of being physically present in the virtual world through special devices, and interactive, because users can interact with the virtual environment and the virtual world's response in real time to those actions (e.g., touch things and feel them, very advanced sounds) [19, 20].

VR systems can be classified into three major categories: non-immersive, immersive, and semi-immersive. These categories are based on one of the important features of VR, its immersion-presence, which can influence the effects on the attention of users [21] and the type of interfaces or components utilized in the system [22, 23]. The non-immersive VR system is the least immersive and least expensive of the VR systems, as it requires the least sophisticated components. Although the user is connected to the virtual world, he still has the possibility of communicating with the external environment [22, 24]. The semi-immersive VR system provides high level of immersion, while keeping the simplicity of the desktop VR or utilizing some physical models. An example of such system includes the CAVE (Cave Automatic Virtual Environment), where the users maintain an interaction with the real environment [17, 23]. The immersive VR system is the most expensive and gives the highest level of immersion, most of the times (according to the needs of the user) providing 360° content [25]. The HMD blocks the view of the user from the real environment and can facilitate the attainment of full immersion. Gesture-sensing gloves, synthesized sounds, and vibrotactile platforms allow the stimulation of multiple senses for better interaction with the virtual environment, excluding sights and sounds from the real environment [22, 23, 26, 27].

History of VR

The term VR is relatively a new one, but the same cannot be said about the tool. For the last 60 years, the scientific community has been working on its development. The beginning of what today has widely become known as VR has started back in the 1950s and 1960s. Many inventions were developed before VR, and they helped to pave the way for this technological tool.

Sensorama was the first machine that tried to engage all senses of the users. In 1957, Morton Heilig tried to create a multi-sensory experience via specific components like smell generators and vibrating chairs [28, 29]. In 1961, *Headsight* was developed by Philco Corporation, and it incorporated motion tracking and dual monitor displays for military training purposes. This invention was the first head-mounted display that had been used [30]. After that, its foundations were laid and the great development by Ivan Sutherland in 1965 was pivotal. His doctoral thesis entitled "Sketchpad: a man-machine graphical communication system" was the key to how computers could be used for making interactive graphics. Afterwards, the same investor published the seminar paper "A head-mounted three dimensional display" and developed the Ultimate Display, which showed a greater real-time interaction with VR via the first computer-generated interface [17, 29, 31, 32].

The 1970s and 1980s were a heady time in the field. Optical advances ran parallel to projects that worked on haptic devices and other instruments that allowed you to move around in the virtual space. However, until then, the cost was too high making it only available for powerful governments and for very sophisticated development and research programs. At NASA Ames Research Center in the mid-1980s, for example, the Virtual Interface Environment Workstation (VIEW) system combined a head-mounted device with gloves to enable the haptic interaction. A great use of VR in the 1980s was that it allowed pilots to have many hours of practice in virtual contexts and acquire a high degree of mastery in many diverse circumstances [17, 29, 33, 34].

Even after all of these developments in VR-related areas, there wasn't an all-encompassing term to describe this emerging field. This all changed in 1987 when Jaron Lanier, founder of the visual programming lab (VPL), coined (or according to some popularized) the term "Virtual Reality" [35]. Through his company VPL research, Jaron developed a range of VR gear including the Dataglove (along with Tom Zimmerman) and the EyePhone HMD. They were the first company to sell VR goggles (EyePhone 1 $9400; EyePhone HRX $49,000) and gloves ($9000). After these developments, VR started to gain greater presence in many fields of research and application mainly due to their unique properties [17, 29, 35–37].

In the 1990s, the availability of high performance computers with fast 3D graphics was increased and, as a result, it became feasible to perform nontrivial physical simulations at fully interactive speeds in a Virtual Environment (VE) for the first time [24]. VR systems became available for the consumer market between 1985 and 1990, when several video games companies started to sell quite inexpensive HMD and data gloves, for the public, which used to interact with the virtual worlds [37].

Through the years, better and more advanced virtual environments have been developed which can work in much simpler and economical systems. The evolution of the field has also provided the user to participate in the co-design of such environments and even change between virtual environments during a single intervention. The future possibilities are endless for those involved in this field of technology.

Applications of VR

The technological advances led to the experience of a life-changing world and allowed the development of new user-friendly devices. VR is one of these devices which, because of its settings and functions, can be used in many fields in our daily life. Use of VR technology is growing rapidly in industries such as in medicine and medical technology; military equipment and battle simulations; business and economic modeling; virtual designing and prototyping of cars, heavy equipment, and aircraft; lathe operations; architectural design and simulations; teleoperation of robotics and machinery; athletic and fitness training; airport simulations; equipment stress testing and control; accident investigation and analysis; law enforcement; and hazard detection and prevention [7, 16, 29, 38, 39].

Several studies have demonstrated significant results in the application of VR programs in medicine. There is a vast array of potential uses for VR in the clinic, including for the purposes of diagnosing psychiatric and nervous system disorders, educating patients about medical procedures, and promoting physical and cognitive rehabilitation and function [40–46]. Moreover, in the field of medical training, Varshney et al. [47] found that these high-tech systems play an important role in coaching and allow people to gain expertise in very precise procedures, thus avoiding the risk of training on real patients, such as surgery or biopsy procedures [48]. Also, VR can be used to manage acute and chronic physical pain (i.e., burn injuries, routine medical procedures, dental procedures, cancer pain) [11, 49–53] and treat a variety of psychiatric disorders like anxiety disorders via exposure therapy (acrophobia, aviophobia, arachnophobia, etc.) and eating and substance use disorders via cognitive control training [29, 54–57].

Although the field of clinical technology lacks a strict consensus regarding the definition of VR and which specific technologies fall under it, VR broadly offers the possibility of creating therapeutic environments for the assessment and treatment of medical conditions. Many studies have provided evidence that the use of VR as a clinical tool is not only beneficial but will become an actuality in healthcare, and nurse researchers will need to evaluate nursing applications for this technology.

Virtual Reality and Symptoms Management

Virtual Reality (VR) is one of the strategies which have been identified as a cognitive-behavioral intervention. These interventions are thought to affect symptoms by changing symptom-related thoughts, diminishing those beliefs that exacerbate symptoms, and increasing personal perceptions of control over symptoms [52, 58–60].

Many studies have been done regarding the effectiveness of VR in the clinical context and symptoms management in different diseases. These include physical and/or psychological symptoms. In 1992, the first clinical experiment was conducted to explore the effectiveness of VE desensitization in the treatment of agoraphobia (i.e., fear of being in places or situations from which escape might be difficult or embarrassing). Findings showed that the group that received VR treatment exhibited a significant decrease in agoraphobia symptoms (i.e., anxiety, stress) [61, 62].

A study by Ryu et al. [63], where they utilized a gaming VR intervention in children undergoing elective day surgery and general anesthesia, showed that children who used VR gaming had lower pre-treating anxiety than those who did not use VR. Moreover, Dehghan et al. investigated the effect of VR technology on preoperative anxiety in 40 children using a Solomon four-group randomized clinical trial and found that anxiety of children reduced [64]. Krijn et al. [65] explored that VR was more effective compared to control (no intervention) in patients with acrophobia, while Aminabadi et al. [66] found that there was a significant decrease in state anxiety scores ($p < 0.001$) with the use of VR in children during dental procedures. Song and Park [67] determined the effects of training using VR games on balance and gait ability, as well as the psychological characteristics of stroke patients, such as depression and interpersonal relationships, by comparing them with the effects of ergometer training. The group with the VR showed more significant improvement in their depression state after the intervention, than the group with ergometer training. Moreover, Schneider et al. [68–70] found that VR decreased the mean state of anxiety in cancer patients during the chemotherapy session. Mosadeghi and colleagues [71], who published the first study in which they evaluated the acceptability and feasibility of VR in a diverse cohort of 30 hospitalized patients, found that after a single use of an immersive, HMD VR intervention, 61% of the patients reported significant improvements in their mood.

Within the field of posttraumatic stress disorder (PTSD), Rothbaum and Mellman [72] conducted a study where they exposed a sample of ten combat veterans with PTSD into two environments: a virtual Huey helicopter flying over a virtual representation of Vietnam and a clearing surrounded by the jungle. All the patients interviewed after the 6-month follow-up period reported reductions in PTSD symptoms (i.e., anxiety, depression, stress) ranging from 15% to 67%.

Numerous reports have documented the potential analgesic effect of immersive VR in various medical settings including cancer therapy [73–75], dental care [76], and transurethral prostate ablation [77]. Many studies referred to the use of VR during wound dressing changes as part of burn care. In 2000, Hoffman et al. [78] found that in a sample of 12 adults and children, there was a better pain control during wound dressing changes and physical therapy when experiencing the environment created by HMD in VR rather than video games graphics. Similarly other researchers [79–83] utilized VR as a distraction intervention during wound dressing changes of burn injuries in children and adults and they found statistically significant reductions of pain rates during and after using the VR intervention. Frere et al. [84] who used a crossover design with 25 persons to test the distracting qualities of a HMD during dental prophylaxis found that fear and pain were reduced significantly during the distraction condition. Same results were found in Aminabadi et al. [66] study who also found that in a group of 120 children there was a significant decrease in pain perception ($p < 0.001$) and state anxiety scores ($p < 0.001$) with the use of virtual reality eyeglasses during dental treatment. More recently, Gerceker et al. [85] evaluated pain rate during intravenous phlebotomy in 121 children and stated that pain scores were determined to be lower in the group with VR rather than the control group. Furthermore, in other studies with children, VR was applied during port access for chemotherapy treatment and found that there was a significant difference on pain and fear for the procedure of treatment and parents mentioned that the intervention as a distracter was effective in diverting their child's attention [21, 75, 86].

In the rehabilitation and functional field, a review of Rose et al. [40] investigated the studies that utilized VR in the assessment and rehabilitation of specific disabilities resulting from brain injury, including executive dysfunction, memory impairments, spatial ability impairments, attention deficits, and unilateral visual neglect. They found that the use of VR in brain damage rehabilitation is expanding dramatically and will become an integral part of cognitive assessment and rehabilitation in the future. Cho et al. [87] found that ten stroke patients significantly improved in conventional behavioral tests after training and that there was an effect after the use of VR to recover the proprioception (i.e., kinesthesia). Moreover, Garcia et al. [88] and Plancher et al. [89] worked with patients with Alzheimer's disease and found that VR can help them in cognitive rehabilitation and improve their quality of life. Finally, in their study with Parkinson's disease patients, Lee et al. [90] provided evidence that the balance, activities of daily living, and depressive disorder status significantly differed between, before, and after treatment in the experimental group, and significantly differed between the experimental group and control group, after using VR dance exercise.

VR effect has also been demonstrated for physical symptoms. For example, the effect of VR has been studied in cancer patients experiencing chemotherapy-related symptoms such as nausea, vomiting, anorexia, and fatigue. Kaneda et al. [91] used immersive VR during chemotherapy treatment in ten adults and found that nausea and vomiting improved for all patients. The majority of patients also reported lower anxiety levels as they focused their attention on the VR environment. Two studies [68, 70] with cancer patients demonstrated a statistically significant difference in fatigue (i.e., reduction) immediately after chemotherapy treatment when subjects used the VR intervention. Cho and Sohng [87] in their study with hemodialysis patients with end-stage renal failure found a statistically significant decrease of fatigue at the intervention group with VR exercise program while almost no changes were noted in the control group. In a recent systematic literature review [92], identified 15 studies where Virtual Reality applications have been utilized to manage pain and fatigue. this demonstrates the emerging value of VR in the management of physical symptoms.

Augmented Reality

What Is AR?

Augmented reality (AR) is a technology that uses a computer-generated virtual imagery information to augment/enhance a live real-time direct or indirect real-world environment. Sometimes, this is referred to as "mixed reality" or "blended reality" [93, 94].

AR utilizes some aspects of VR and it is as a prolongation of VR. It is different from VR from which the user is completely immersed in a computer-generated virtual environment. However, AR uses minimal interference, allowing virtual presences to be blended into users reality rather than removing them from it [95]. AR enhances the perceived effect of integrating virtual information or objects into a real-world environment via computer-generated images, objects, information or scenes, and interaction to enhance the perception [96, 97]. In other words, the target of AR is not to establish a fully artificial environment but to cover images produced from a computer onto images of the real world [98]. Therefore, it uses machines which allow users to view the surrounding real environment but enhanced with virtual images. Some devices that can be employed as hardware for running applications of AR are tablets, mobile phones, and AR glasses [99].

Azuma et al. [96, 100] supplied three commonly accepted criteria that characterized AR systems as technologies that [101] combine real and virtual environments, are interactive in real time, and indicated in three dimensions. So, the fundamental idea of AR is to combine or mix the view of the real environment with additional virtual content. This virtual content can appeal to different senses such as sight, hearing, touch, and smell [100, 102].

AR Technology

From the point of view of technology devices, AR can be defined as a set of techniques and tools that allow adding information to physical reality. Three characteristics describe the AR technology: "combining virtual reality with real world," "real-time interaction," and "essential 3D space." A computer device is needed in order to connect virtual content to the real world. This device provides a window (display) through which the physical world can be seen. As regards the projection displays, the virtual elements are projected on the real objects in order to be augmented. A single room-mounted projector is used in order the projection can occur, without any display system the head of the user. A virtual image is generated by the projector on the room surface using an automated calibration procedure that takes into account the structure of the surface overlapping the virtual image. Furthermore, a software application is necessary to be on the computer (AR platform) in order for the virtual components to be visible in the display, as an augmentation to reality. Marker-based and markerless systems are the two main software applications used in AR system. In the AR marker-based systems, the computer webcam recognizes the stylized pictures, which are black and white, which are superimposed in real-time multimedia contents: video, audio, 3D objects, and so forth. Instead, in the markerless AR systems the software application uses a GPS and compass device in order to find the position and orientation of the user and add the virtual contents in an accurate position on or in the real environment. Moreover, glasses are a tool that most AR hardware use which project virtual 3D images onto the real environment. The first developed glasses were Google Glass and Epson Smart Glasses, while the newer devices combine AR glasses with a system of tracking cameras and sensors. While the camera captures the physical world, virtual structures are added in the screen. An example of a new device is the HoloLens which is created by Microsoft and offers the same immersive experience of HMDs, but the physical reality is present to the users [98, 103, 104].

There are many different hardware devices that can be used for AR. Handheld devices, display system worn by the user (non-handheld devices), and projection displays are some of the technologies that are used in AR rendering. Smartphones and tablets are the most commonly used handheld devices, which include a camera and sensors such as accelerometer, Global Positioning System (GPS), and solid-state compass. These characteristics make them a suitable AR platform which takes in real time the surrounding environment and the virtual elements are overlay to the real world [103].

HMD is a non-handheld device, which users wear it on their head such as a helmet or glasses. HMD's advantage is that the display stays in front of the eyes, no matter what direction the user might look, supporting situation awareness, and the users have no connection with the real environment. An example of a HMD is Google Glass which is used by the Radboud University Medical Center, Nijmegen, and the Academic Medical Center, Amsterdam, to explore the possible added value for healthcare and medical education.

History of AR

Historically, the term Augmented Reality was established in 1990, but the development of AR starts in the 1960s. In the 1960s, VR system was also developed by Ivan Sutherland at Harvard University and the University of Utah [95]. In 1972, Alan Kay proposed the first conceptual tablet computer, named the Dynabook. The Dynabook is probably recognized as being the precursor of the tablet computers decades before the iPad [105].

In the early 1990s, Tom Caudell and David Mizell developed the term "augmented reality" to refer to overlaying computer-presented material on top of the real world. Two advantages of AR compared to VR is that AR requires less processing power since less pixels have to be rendered, as Caudell and Mizell pointed. Also, they acknowledged the increased registration requirements in order to align real and virtual [106].

In 1994, Paul Milgram and Fumio Kishino wrote their seminal paper "Taxonomy of Mixed Reality Visual Displays" in which they described the Reality-Virtuality Continuum. This continuum spans from the real environment to the virtual environment. In between there are Augmented Reality, closer to the real environment, and Augmented Virtuality, which is closer to the virtual environment [5]. Today, Augmented Reality is commonly described by Milgram's Continuum and Azuma's definition [96].

After 2000, the increase in the use of AR came along with the technological advances that made it available and useful. Since this first creation, AR has been developed further in a variety of fields with a numerous applications.

Applications of AR

Nowadays, AR is used widely in many fields. An example of the use of AR in entertainment is its application in many movies. The most widely used examples include the "Minority Report" (starring Tom Cruise), the "Iron Man" (starring Robert Downey Jr), with more recent examples to include "Creative Control" (starring

Benjamin Dickinson) and "Valerian and the City of a Thousand Planets" (starring Dane DeHaan) just to report a few. Moreover, this technology is used by Pokémon Go, an application game in smartphones, which was based on the geo-location service LBS (location-based services) AR, where smartphones are held by the players. With GPS positioning, map information was presented based on LBS technology, displaying the player's geographic location in real time, combined with the AR technology. In the player's mobile phones' screen, they could see the virtual Pokémon (through the camera lens) additionally to the real environment, which was superimposed on the virtual environment in the virtual object [6].

AR, while not necessarily a new technology, is becoming more well known and gaining some momentum in healthcare. Some applications of AR in the clinical setting mainly include surgery, medical rehabilitation, medical consultation, medical diagnosis, and medical education and training [107].

The first virtual system in medicine was introduced by Robert Mann in the mid-1960s. This system was utilized as a tool to optimally select the most appropriate procedure for orthopedic diseases. Another application of the system included its use as a new training environment for orthopedic residents. The range of applications for VR and AR systems within the medical context was expanded with the introduction of wearable devices [108].

In the medical education field, the first applications were some on hands-on procedures which appeared over a decade later [109]. AR has the potential to provide powerful, contextual, and situated learning experiences, as well as to aid exploration of the complex interconnections seen in information in the real world. Examples of these applications in medical education include representation of mechanisms in space and time dimensions in physiology, or 4D; and 3D visualizations of difficult structures in anatomy. AR can be used by students to construct new understanding based upon their interactions with virtual objects, which bring underlying data to life. Environmental sciences, ecosystems, language, chemistry, geography, and history are some disciplines in higher education where AR can be applied [110, 111]. An acceptable application of AR is in clinical care because it provides doctors with an internal view of the patient, without the need for invasive procedures [99].

Augmented Reality and Symptoms Management

The clinical care context is a complex one that often creates a stressful and demanding environment for students but also for medical professionals. The possibility to train under simulated conditions through AR systems that mirror the real environment is a valuable tool for healthcare professionals' training (e.g., training to treat rare conditions) and one that safeguards patient safety. The positive effects of AR are not limited to improving education and training, but it can also lead to better outcomes in patient care. One way that patient care outcomes can be improved through AR application is with an improved symptom management [94, 112]. Despite AR potential in this field there are only a limited number of studies that have been done in clinical conditions in order to determine the AR efficacy for specific symptoms management. Several studies were done studying different systems of AR technology in many different cases of patients [107].

A promising use of AR includes its application as a tool management during painful procedures. Mott et al. [113] tested the efficacy of AR in 42 children (age 3–14 years) with acute burns and a total burn surface area ranging from 1% to 16%. AR was compared to Cognitive Behavioral Therapy (CBT) techniques (e.g., distraction, breathing, positive reinforcement) as an adjunct to analgesia and sedation during dressing changes. The effectiveness of the intervention was measured against pain scores, pulse rates (PR), respiratory rates (RR), and oxygen saturations (SaO$_2$) that were recorded pre-procedurally, at 10 min intervals, and post-procedurally. Mean pain scores were significantly lower ($p = 0.0060$) in the AR group compared to the control group. Respiratory and pulse rates showed significant changes over time within groups; however, these were not significantly different between the two study groups.

AR technology can also be used for the phantom limb pain treatment [114]. Phantom limb pain refers to patients who have lost part of their limbs but they can still feel it present or feel the pains of their amputated limbs [115]. The implementation of AR technology helps amputees to see the virtual limp appear on the screen. When the patient moves the amputated limp, the screen will show the virtual limp with the same action, through the interactions to activate and allow the patient to control the originally amputated limb with their brain, in order to achieve a therapeutic effect [116]. A systematic review [117] introduced studies comparing AR with VR and conventional therapies for the treatment of the phantom limb pain. The study showed that the AR approach provided better results, especially in terms of providing a more realistic simulation. The proposed system, with the use of a standard computer and webcam, provides the possibility to the patient to independently practice daily at home. The AR technology provides a highly controllable environment with tasks of different difficulty levels to the patients allowing them to perform the exercise gradually and systematically. Desmond et al. [118] tested three patients with a mirror therapy approach based on AR, comparing the results with the classic mirror box. Instead of using a HMD for the AR, they used a simple screen with a consequent loss in terms of immersion. The two approaches had similar results, with the exception of a rather vivid sensation experienced by patients when the AR was used to display unexpected or abnormal movements. It is argued that AR technology offers a promising new approach to the investigation of phantom experience and potentially to the treatment of phantom pain. Moreover, Bach et al. [119] developed an AR prototype consisting of a HMD and a stereo camera system. This AR system allowed recording images of the healthy patient's hand, processing the images in real time to create a reproduction of the missing hand, and finally displaying the virtual hand at the place of the missing one. Unfortunately, the authors did not present any study concerning the use of their system with patients. In a case study by Ortiz-Catalan et al. [120], they explored a treatment in which the virtual limb responded directly to myoelectric activity at the stump, while the illusion of a restored limb was enhanced through AR. The proposed set of technologies was administered to a chronic Phantom Limp Pain patient who has shown resistance to a variety of treatments (including mirror therapy) for 48 years. Individual and simultaneous phantom movements were predicted using myoelectric pattern recognition and were then used as input for VR and AR environments, as well as for a racing game. Finally, the patient reported a gradual reduction of sustained level of pain to complete pain-free periods. Ortiz-Catalan et al. [116], in a sample of 14 patients with intractable chronic phantom limb pain, introduced 12 sessions of phantom motor execution using machine learning, augmented and virtual reality, and serious gaming. Phantom limb pain decreased from pre-treatment to the last treatment session by 47% (SD 39; absolute mean change 1.0 [0.8]; $p = 0.001$) for weighted pain distribution, 32% (38; absolute mean change 1.6 [1.8]; $p = 0.007$) for the numeric rating scale, and 51% (33; absolute mean change 9.6 [8.1]; $p = 0.0001$) for the pain rating index. The numeric rating scale score for intrusion of phantom limb pain in activities of daily living and sleep was reduced by 43% (SD 37; absolute mean change 2.4 [2.3]; $p = 0.004$) and 61% (39; absolute mean change 2.3 [1.8]; $p = 0.001$), respectively. Two out of four patients who were on medication reduced their intake by 81% (i.e., absolute reduction 1300 mg, gabapentin) and 33% (absolute reduction 75 mg, pregabalin). It is important to note that the effect of the intervention remained 6 months after the last treatment.

AR technology has also been utilized in rehabilitation cases. Lee, Kim, and Lee [121] determined the effects of AR-based postural control training on balance and gait function in 21 stroke patients who were assigned to either an experimental group ($n = 10$) or a control group ($n = 11$). Patients in both groups received a general physical therapy program for a duration of 30 min per session, 5 days per week, for a period of 4 weeks. Participants in the experimental group received additional AR-based postural control training for 30 min per day, 3 days per week, for a period of 4 weeks. Results of repeated-measures analysis of covariance showed a significant main effect of time on timed up-and-go test, Berg Balance Scale, velocity, cadence, step length and stride length of paretic and non-paretic sides. In addition, walking velocity, step length, and stride length on both the paretic and non-paretic sides showed a significant group time interaction effect. The results of this study provided evidence in support of incorporating an AR environment to help stoke patients into postural control training for improving their gait.

Voss et al. [122] developed a system for automatic facial expression recognition, which runs on Google Glass and delivers real-time social cues to the user. They evaluated this system in children with autism spectrum disorder (ASD) and used it as a behavioral aid. These children, in contrast with neuro-typically developing children, can greatly benefit from real-time noninvasive emotional cues and are more sensitive to sensory input. Their initial findings had shown that SuperpowerGlass can be an effective tool for delivering real-time emotion cues to a user, particularly for children with ASD.

AR has also been presented as an effective technology for treating phobias and anxiety. However, to our knowledge, the sense of presence and anxiety has not been compared in AR and VR systems that include acrophobic scenarios. The equivalence of AR and VR for presence and anxiety measures could be potentially important for a major application area of virtual environment technology. Juan et al. [123] and Botella et al. [124] presented the first AR system for the treatment of phobias of cockroaches and spiders. In these works, they demonstrated that, with a single 1-h session, patients significantly reduced their fear and avoidance. Initially, the system was tested in a case study [124], and then it was tested on nine patients suffering from phobia of small animals [123]. For the treatment of acrophobia, Juan et al. [125] also proposed the use of immersive photography in an AR system. In this system, 41 participants without acrophobia walked around at the top of a staircase in a real environment and in an immersive photography environment. Immediately after their experience, the participants were given the SUS questionnaire to assess their subjective sense of presence. The users' scores in the immersive photography environment were very high. However, statistically significant differences were found between the real and immersive photography environments. Juan and David [126] developed an AR system and a VR system that included acrophobic scenarios. Twenty non-phobic users used both systems in order to compare the levels of presence and anxiety. For the anxiety level, the results showed that there is a significant difference between the anxiety level before starting the intervention and the anxiety level during the different stages of the intervention. After the correlation between anxiety and presence, results showed a very low correlation between anxiety and presence. These results suggested that AR is likely to be as effective as VR in treating acrophobia, but they believed that AR can be used as an alternative for treating acrophobia based on the results. Yeh et al. [127] in their study explored the effects of VR and AR in the treatment of claustrophobia. They investigated the potential effects of each intervention on induced anxiety in 34 individuals. AR and VR have induced anxiety, which was reflected in the subjective and objective physiological indicators. However, no significant difference was found in the effects of AR and VR on the induced anxiety. Wirzeslen et al. [128–130] studied the preliminary results of the level of anxiety in a comparative analysis of AR and VE applied to the treatment of patients with cockroach and spider phobia or healthy volunteers. The three studies found a statistically significant decrease of anxiety after the intervention of AR.

Conclusion

The emergence of exciting new technologies, such as VR and AR systems, provides endless opportunities for healthcare innovation in a range of key areas. Despite their relatively recent utilization in healthcare, their continual improvement (e.g., user-friendly, noninvasive, and low cost) has opened up new possibilities for a diversity of applications. The chapter summarized the potential importance and possibilities that VR and AR can bring to healthcare, as an adjuvant tool to professional engagement as well as to patient care and especially on symptoms management. Increasing the use of these techniques in healthcare interventions can contribute to improved outcomes, particularly in health prevention strategies and in chronic care settings.

Healthcare professionals should consider developing and applying these technologies in the management of many symptoms. Personalization of these interventions that focus on the needs of individuals may help to provide a greater sense of control and may be helpful to motivate individuals to decrease and manage their symptoms more effectively. Healthcare professionals may find it helpful to use VR and AR and personalize these as part of a patient-centered, goal-oriented care planning activity.

References

 1. Hsieh M, Lee J. Preliminary study of VR and AR applications in medical and healthcare education. J Nurs Health Stud. 2018;3(1):1.
 2. Pantelidis P, Chorti A, Papagiouvanni I, Paparoidamis G, Drosos C, Panagiotakopoulos T, et al. Virtual and augmented reality in medical education. In: Medical and surgical education–past, present and future. London: IntechOpen; 2018. p. 77–97.
 3. Corbett-Davies S, et al. An advanced interaction framework for augmented reality based exposure treatment. In: 2013 IEEE Virtual Reality (VR). Washington, DC: IEEE; 2013.
 4. Milgram P, et al. Augmented reality: a class of displays on the reality-virtuality continuum. In: Telemanipulator and telepresence technologies. Bellingham: International Society for Optics and Photonics; 1995.
 5. Milgram P, Kishino F. A taxonomy of mixed reality visual displays. IEICE Trans Inf Syst. 1994;77(12):1321–9.
 6. Hsieh MC, Huang KY. Augmented reality is so fun! A new technology application combining virtuality and reality. Taiwan: ROC; 2016.
 7. Wexelblat A. Virtual reality: applications and explorations. New York, NY: Academic Press; 2014.
 8. Ferguson C, Davidson PM, Scott PJ, Jackson D, Hickman LD. Augmented reality, virtual reality and gaming: an integral part of nursing. Contemp Nurse. 2015;51:1.
 9. Conn C, et al. Virtual environments and interactivity: windows to the future. In: ACM SIGGRAPH 89 Panel Proceedings. New York, NY: ACM; 1989.
10. Biocca F. Virtual reality technology: a tutorial. J Commun. 1992;42(4):23–72.
11. Wiederhold MD, Wiederhold BK. Virtual reality and interactive simulation for pain distraction. Pain Med. 2007;8:S182.
12. Rubino F, Soler L, Marescaux J, Maisonneuve H. Advances in virtual reality are wide ranging. BMJ. 2002;324(7337):612.
13. McCloy R, Stone R. Science, medicine, and the future. Virtual reality in surgery. BMJ. 2001;323(7318):912–5.
14. Szekely G, Satava RM. Virtual reality in medicine. Interview by Judy Jones. BMJ. 1999;319(7220):1305.
15. ABCT. Applications and issues for the use of virtual reality technology for cognitive/behavioral/neuro-psychological assessment and intervention. In: Workshop presented at the 34th Annual Convention of the Association for Advancement of Behavior Therapy. New York, NY: ABCT; 2000.
16. Ausburn LJ, Ausburn FB. Desktop virtual reality: a powerful new technology for teaching and research in industrial teacher education. J Ind Teach Educ. 2004;41(4):1–16.
17. Mandal S. Brief introduction of virtual reality & its challenges. Int J Sci Eng Res. 2013;4(4):304–9.
18. Napolitano MA, Hayes S, Russo G, Muresu D, Giordano A, Foster GD. Using avatars to model weight loss behaviors: participant attitudes and technology development. J Diabetes Sci Technol. 2013;7(4):1057–65.

19. Liszio S, Graf L, Masuch M. The relaxing effect of virtual nature: immersive technology provides relief in acute stress situations. Annu Rev Cyberther Telemed. 2018;16:87.
20. Yu C, Lee H, Luo X. The effect of virtual reality forest and urban environments on physiological and psychological responses. Urban For Urban Green. 2018;35:106–14.
21. Nilsson S, Finnström B, Kokinsky E, Enskär K. The use of Virtual Reality for needle-related procedural pain and distress in children and adolescents in a paediatric oncology unit. Eur J Oncol Nurs. 2009;13(2):102–9.
22. Bamodu O, Ye XM. Virtual reality and virtual reality system components. In: Advanced materials research. Stafa-Zurich: Trans Tech Publ; 2013.
23. Brooks FP. What's real about virtual reality? IEEE Comput Graph Appl. 1999;19(6):16–27.
24. Chirico A, Lucidi F, De Laurentiis M, Milanese C, Napoli A, Giordano A. Virtual reality in health system: beyond entertainment. a mini-review on the efficacy of VR during cancer treatment. J Cell Physiol. 2016;231(2):275–87.
25. Meehan M, et al. Physiological measures of presence in stressful virtual environments. In: ACM Transactions on Graphics (tog). New York, NY: ACM; 2002.
26. Hoffman HG, Patterson DR, Seibel E, Soltani M, Jewett-Leahy L, Sharar SR. Virtual reality pain control during burn wound debridement in the hydrotank. Clin J Pain. 2008;24(4):299–304.
27. Maples-Keller JL, Bunnell BE, Kim SJ, Rothbaum BO. The use of virtual reality technology in the treatment of anxiety and other psychiatric disorders. Harv Rev Psychiatry. 2017;25(3):103–13.
28. Dinh HQ, et al. Evaluating the importance of multi-sensory input on memory and the sense of presence in virtual environments. In: Proceedings IEEE Virtual Reality (Cat. No. 99CB36316). Washington, DC: IEEE; 1999.
29. Onyesolu MO, Eze FU. Understanding virtual reality technology: advances and applications. In: Advances in computer science engineering. London: IntechOpen; 2011. p. 53–70.
30. Comeau C. Headsight television system provides remote surveillance. Electronics. 1961;10:86–90.
31. Sutherland IE. A head-mounted three dimensional display. In: Proceedings of the December 9-11, 1968, Fall Joint Computer Conference, Part I. New York, NY: ACM; 1968.
32. Sutherland IE. The ultimate display. In: Multimedia: from Wagner to virtual reality; 1965. p. 506–8.
33. Stone RJ. Haptic feedback: a brief history from telepresence to virtual reality. In: International Workshop on Haptic Human-Computer Interaction. Cham: Springer; 2000.
34. The Franklin Institute. History of virtual reality. 2019. https://www.fi.edu/virtual-reality/history-of-virtual-reality.
35. Conn C, Lanier J, Minsky M, Fisher S, Druin A. Virtual environments and interactivity: windows to the future. ACM Siggr Comput Graph. 1989;23(5):7–18.
36. Gorini A, Riva G, Deacon G, Kobak R, et al. Virtual reality in anxiety disorders: the past and the future. Expert Rev Neurother. 2008;8(2):215–33.
37. Virtual Reality Society. History of virtual reality. 2017. https://www.vrs.org.uk/virtual-reality/history.html.
38. Greenleaf W, Piantanida T. Medical applications of virtual reality technology. In: The biomedical engineering handbook. Boca Raton, FL: CRC Press; 2000.
39. Whyte J. Industrial applications of virtual reality in architecture and construction. J Inf Technol Construct. 2003;8(4):43–50.
40. Rose FD, Brooks BM, Rizzo AA. Virtual reality in brain damage rehabilitation. CyberPsychol Behav. 2005;8(3):241–62.
41. Holden MK. Virtual environments for motor rehabilitation. CyberPsychol Behav. 2005;8(3):187–211.
42. Cherniack EP. Not just fun and games: applications of virtual reality in the identification and rehabilitation of cognitive disorders of the elderly. Disab Rehabil Assist Technol. 2011;6(4):283–9.

43. Hanten G, Cook L, Orsten K, Chapman SB, Li X, Wilde EA, et al. Effects of traumatic brain injury on a virtual reality social problem solving task and relations to cortical thickness in adolescence. Neuropsychologia. 2011;49(3):486–97.
44. Yip BC, Man DW. Virtual reality-based prospective memory training program for people with acquired brain injury. NeuroRehabilitation. 2013;32(1):103–15.
45. Wang M, Reid D. Using the virtual reality-cognitive rehabilitation approach to improve contextual processing in children with autism. Sci World J. 2013;2013:716890.
46. Jimenez YA, Lewis SJ. Radiation therapy patient education using VERT: combination of technology with human care. J Med Radiat Sci. 2018;65(2):158–62.
47. Varshney R, Frenkiel S, Nguyen LH, Young M, Del Maestro R, Zeitouni A, et al. Development of the McGill simulator for endoscopic sinus surgery: a new high-fidelity virtual reality simulator for endoscopic sinus surgery. Am J Rhinol Allergy. 2014;28(4):330–4.
48. Danforth DR, Procter M, Chen R, Johnson M, Heller R. Development of virtual patient simulations for medical education. J Virt Worlds Res. 2009;2(2):1.
49. Parsons TD, Rizzo AA. Affective outcomes of virtual reality exposure therapy for anxiety and specific phobias: a meta-analysis. J Behav Ther Exp Psychiatry. 2008;39(3):250–61.
50. Mahrer NE, Gold JI. The use of virtual reality for pain control: a review. Curr Pain Headache Rep. 2009;13(2):100–9.
51. Morris LD, Louw QA, Grimmer-Somers K. The effectiveness of virtual reality on reducing pain and anxiety in burn injury patients: a systematic review. Clin J Pain. 2009;25(9):815–26.
52. Malloy KM, Milling LS. The effectiveness of virtual reality distraction for pain reduction: a systematic review. Clin Psychol Rev. 2010;30(8):1011–8.
53. Gordon EM, Li BM, Liu S, Chawla SP, Liu SM, Liu SM. RELAX: an immersion virtual reality relaxation intervention for quality of life improvement in cancer patients. J Clin Oncol. 2018;36:152.
54. Botella C, Quero S, Baños RM, Perpiña C, Garcia-Palacios A, Riva G. Virtual reality and psychotherapy. Cybertherapy. 2004;99:37–52.
55. Ferrer-García M, Gutiérrez-Maldonado J. The use of virtual reality in the study, assessment, and treatment of body image in eating disorders and nonclinical samples: a review of the literature. Body Image. 2012;9(1):1–11.
56. Hone-Blanchet A, Wensing T, Fecteau S. The use of virtual reality in craving assessment and cue-exposure therapy in substance use disorders. Front Hum Neurosci. 2014;8:844.
57. van Bennekom MJ, de Koning PP, Denys D. Virtual reality objectifies the diagnosis of psychiatric disorders: a literature review. Front Psychiatry. 2017;8:163.
58. Anderson KO, Cohen MZ, Mendoza TR, Guo H, Harle MT, Cleeland CS. Brief cognitive-behavioral audiotape interventions for cancer-related pain: immediate but not long-term effectiveness. Cancer. 2006;107(1):207–14.
59. Kwekkeboom KL, Kneip J, Pearson L. A pilot study to predict success with guided imagery for cancer pain. Pain Manag Nurs. 2003;4(3):112–23.
60. Kwekkeboom KL, Abbott-Anderson K, Wanta B. Feasibility of a patient-controlled cognitive-behavioral intervention for pain, fatigue, and sleep disturbance in cancer. Oncol Nurs Forum. 2010;37(3):E151–9.
61. North MM, North SM, Coble JR. Effectiveness of virtual environment desensitization in the treatment of agoraphobia. Pres Teleoper Virt Environ. 1996;5(3):346–52.
62. North MM, North SM, Coble JR, Pyle T, Wilson A. Virtual reality therapy: an innovative paradigm. Vienna: Ipi Press; 1996.
63. Ryu J, Park J, Nahm FS, Jeon Y, Oh A, Lee HJ, et al. The effect of gamification through a virtual reality on preoperative anxiety in pediatric patients undergoing general anesthesia: a prospective, randomized, and controlled trial. J Clin Med. 2018;7(9):284.
64. Dehghan F, Jalali R, Bashiri H. The effect of virtual reality technology on preoperative anxiety in children: a Solomon four-group randomized clinical trial. Perioper Med. 2019;8(1):5.

65. Krijn M, Emmelkamp PM, Biemond R, de Ligny CW, Schuemie MJ, van der Mast, Charles APG. Treatment of acrophobia in virtual reality: the role of immersion and presence. Behav Res Ther. 2004;42(2):229–39.
66. Asl Aminabadi N, Erfanparast L, Sohrabi A, Ghertasi Oskouei S, Naghili A. The impact of virtual reality distraction on pain and anxiety during dental treatment in 4-6 year-old children: a randomized controlled clinical trial. J Dent Res Dent Clin Dent Prospects. 2012;6(4):117–24.
67. bin Song G, cho Park E. Effect of virtual reality games on stroke patients' balance, gait, depression, and interpersonal relationships. J Phys Ther Sci. 2015;27(7):2057–60.
68. Schneider SM, Ellis M, Coombs WT, Shonkwiler EL, Folsom LC. Virtual reality intervention for older women with breast cancer. CyberPsychol Behav. 2003;6(3):301–7.
69. Schneider SM, et al. Virtual reality as a distraction intervention for women receiving chemotherapy. Oncol Nurs Forum. 2004;31:81.
70. Schneider SM, Hood LE. Virtual reality: a distraction intervention for chemotherapy. Oncol Nurs Forum. 2007;34(1):39–46.
71. Mosadeghi S, Reid MW, Martinez B, Rosen BT, Spiegel BMR. Feasibility of an immersive virtual reality intervention for hospitalized patients: an observational cohort study. JMIR Mental Health. 2016;3(2):e28.
72. Rothbaum BO, Mellman TA. Dreams and exposure therapy in PTSD. J Trauma Stress. 2001;14(3):481–90.
73. Gershon J, Zimand E, Pickering M, Rothbaum BO, Hodges L. A pilot and feasibility study of virtual reality as a distraction for children with cancer. J Am Acad Child Adolesc Psychiatry. 2004;43(10):1243–9.
74. Gershon J, Zimand E, Lemos R, Rothbaum BO, Hodges L. Use of virtual reality as a distractor for painful procedures in a patient with pediatric cancer: a case study. CyberPsychol Behav. 2003;6(6):657–61.
75. Windich-Biermeier A, Sjoberg I, Dale JC, Eshelman D, Guzzetta CE. Effects of distraction on pain, fear, and distress during venous port access and venipuncture in children and adolescents with cancer. J Pediatr Oncol Nurs. 2007;24(1):8–19.
76. Hoffman HG, Garcia-Palacios A, Patterson DR, Jensen M, Furness T III, Ammons WF Jr. The effectiveness of virtual reality for dental pain control: a case study. CyberPsychol Behav. 2001;4(4):527–35.
77. Wright JL, Hoffman HG, Sweet RM. Virtual reality as an adjunctive pain control during transurethral microwave thermotherapy. Urology. 2005;66(6):1320.e1–3.
78. Hoffman HG, Patterson DR, Carrougher GJ. Use of virtual reality for adjunctive treatment of adult burn pain during physical therapy: a controlled study. Clin J Pain. 2000;16(3):244–50.
79. Schmitt YS, Hoffman HG, Blough DK, Patterson DR, Jensen MP, Soltani M, et al. A randomized, controlled trial of immersive virtual reality analgesia, during physical therapy for pediatric burns. Burns. 2011;37(1):61–8.
80. Maani CV, Hoffman HG, Morrow M, Maiers A, Gaylord K, McGhee LL, et al. Virtual reality pain control during burn wound debridement of combat-related burn injuries using robot-like arm mounted VR goggles. J Trauma. 2011;71(1 Suppl):S125–30.
81. Carrougher GJ, Hoffman HG, Nakamura D, Lezotte D, Soltani M, Leahy L, et al. The effect of virtual reality on pain and range of motion in adults with burn injuries. J Burn Care Res. 2009;30(5):785–91.
82. van Twillert B, Bremer M, Faber AW. Computer-generated virtual reality to control pain and anxiety in pediatric and adult burn patients during wound dressing changes. J Burn Care Res. 2007;28(5):694–702.
83. Das DA, Grimmer KA, Sparnon AL, McRae SE, Thomas BH. The efficacy of playing a virtual reality game in modulating pain for children with acute burn injuries: a randomized controlled trial [ISRCTN87413556]. BMC Pediatr. 2005;5(1):1.
84. Frere CL, Crout R, Yorty J, McNeil DW. Effects of audiovisual distraction during dental prophylaxis. J Am Dent Assoc. 2001;132(7):1031–8.

85. Gerçeker GÖ, Binay Ş, Bilsin E, Kahraman A, Yılmaz HB. Effects of virtual reality and external cold and vibration on pain in 7-to 12-year-old children during phlebotomy: a randomized controlled trial. J PeriAnesth Nurs. 2018;33(6):981–9.
86. Wolitzky K, Fivush R, Zimand E, Hodges L, Rothbaum BO. Effectiveness of virtual reality distraction during a painful medical procedure in pediatric oncology patients. Psychol Health. 2005;20(6):817–24.
87. Cho H, Sohng K. The effect of a virtual reality exercise program on physical fitness, body composition, and fatigue in hemodialysis patients. J Phys Ther Sci. 2014;26(10):1661–5.
88. Garcia-Betances RI, Jiménez-Mixco V, Arredondo MT, Cabrera-Umpiérrez MF. Using virtual reality for cognitive training of the elderly. Am J Alzheimers Dis Other Dement. 2015;30(1):49–54.
89. Plancher G, Tirard A, Gyselinck V, Nicolas S, Piolino P. Using virtual reality to characterize episodic memory profiles in amnestic mild cognitive impairment and Alzheimer's disease: influence of active and passive encoding. Neuropsychologia. 2012;50(5):592–602.
90. Lee N, Lee D, Song H. Effect of virtual reality dance exercise on the balance, activities of daily living, and depressive disorder status of Parkinson's disease patients. J Phys Ther Sci. 2015;27(1):145–7.
91. VR intervention therapy for emotion related cancer chemotherapy side effects. Int Conf Artif Real Telexistence. 1999.
92. Ioannou A, Papastavrou E, Avraamides MN, Charalambous A. Virtual Reality and Symptoms Management of Anxiety, Depression, Fatigue, and Pain: A Systematic Review. SAGE Open Nursing. January 2020. https://doi.org/10.1177/2377960820936163.
93. Wetzel R, Blum L, Broll W, Oppermann L. Designing mobile augmented reality games. In: Handbook of augmented reality. Cham: Springer; 2011. p. 513–39.
94. Zhu E, Hadadgar A, Masiello I, Zary N. Augmented reality in healthcare education: an integrative review. PeerJ. 2014;2:e469.
95. Van Krevelen D, Poelman R. A survey of augmented reality technologies, applications and limitations. Int J Virtual Real. 2010;9(2):1–20.
96. Azuma RT. A survey of augmented reality. Pres Teleoper Virt Environ. 1997;6(4):355–85.
97. Hugues O, Fuchs P, Nannipieri O. New augmented reality taxonomy: technologies and features of augmented environment. In: Handbook of augmented reality. Berlin: Springer; 2011. p. 47–63.
98. Kamphuis C, Barsom E, Schijven M, Christoph N. Augmented reality in medical education? Perspect Med Educ. 2014;3(4):300–11.
99. Sakakushev BE, Marinov BI, Stefanova PP, Kostianev SS, Georgiou EK. Striving for better medical education: the simulation approach. Folia Med. 2017;59(2):123–31.
100. Azuma R, Baillot Y, Behringer R, Feiner S, Julier S, MacIntyre B. Recent advances in augmented reality. IEEE Comput Graph Appl. 2001;21(6):34–47.
101. Zhou F, et al. Trends in augmented reality tracking, interaction and display: a review of ten years of ISMAR. In: 2008 7th IEEE/ACM International Symposium on Mixed and Augmented Reality. Washington, DC: IEEE; 2008.
102. Yu D, Jin JS, Luo S, Lai W, Huang Q. A useful visualization technique: a literature review for augmented reality and its application, limitation & future direction. In: Visual information communication. New York, NY: Springer; 2009. p. 311–37.
103. Hamacher A, Kim SJ, Cho ST, Pardeshi S, Lee SH, Eun SJ, et al. Application of virtual, augmented, and mixed reality to urology. Int Neurourol J. 2016;20(3):172–81.
104. Genc Y, et al. Marker-less tracking for AR: a learning-based approach. In: Proceedings. International Symposium on Mixed and Augmented Reality. Washington, DC: IEEE; 2002.
105. Goldberg A. Educational uses of a dynabook. Comput Educ. 1979;3(4):247–66.
106. Caudell TP, Mizell DW. Augmented reality: an application of heads-up display technology to manual manufacturing processes. In: Hawaii International Conference on System Sciences. Washington, DC: IEEE; 1992.
107. Herron J. Augmented reality in medical education and training. J Electr Resour Med Lib. 2016;13(2):51–5.

108. Akay M, Marsh A. Virtual reality and its integration into a twenty-first century telemedical information society. 2001.

109. Graur F. Virtual reality in medicine – going beyond the limits. In: The thousand faces of virtual reality. London: IntechOpen; 2014.

110. Johnson L, Levine A, Smith R, Stone S. The 2011 Horizon Report. ERIC. 2011. https://library.educause.edu/resources/2011/2/2011-horizon-report.

111. Klopfer E, Squire K. Environmental detectives – the development of an augmented reality platform for environmental simulations. Educ Technol Res Dev. 2008;56(2):203–28.

112. Chaballout B, Molloy M, Vaughn J, Brisson R III, Shaw R. Feasibility of augmented reality in clinical simulations: using Google glass with manikins. JMIR Med Educ. 2016;2(1):e2.

113. Mott J, Bucolo S, Cuttle L, Mill J, Hilder M, Miller K, et al. The efficacy of an augmented virtual reality system to alleviate pain in children undergoing burns dressing changes: a randomised controlled trial. Burns. 2008;34(6):803–8.

114. Osumi M, Ichinose A, Sumitani M, Wake N, Sano Y, Yozu A, et al. Restoring movement representation and alleviating phantom limb pain through short-term neurorehabilitation with a virtual reality system. Eur J Pain. 2017;21(1):140–7.

115. Weeks SR, Anderson-Barnes VC, Tsao JW. Phantom limb pain: theories and therapies. Neurologist. 2010;16(5):277–86.

116. Ortiz-Catalan M, Guðmundsdóttir RA, Kristoffersen MB, Zepeda-Echavarria A, Caine-Winterberger K, Kulbacka-Ortiz K, et al. Phantom motor execution facilitated by machine learning and augmented reality as treatment for phantom limb pain: a single group, clinical trial in patients with chronic intractable phantom limb pain. Lancet. 2016;388(10062):2885–94.

117. Shen Y. An augmented reality system for hand movement rehabilitation. In: Proceedings of the 2nd International Convention on Rehabilitation Engineering & Assistive Technology. New York, NY: ACM; 2008.

118. Desmond DM, O'Neill K, De Paor A, McDarby G, MacLachlan M. Augmenting the reality of phantom limbs: three case studies using an augmented mirror box procedure. J Prosthet Orthot. 2006;18(3):74–9.

119. Bach F, Schmitz B, Maab H, Cakmak H, Diers M, Bodmann RB, Kamping S, Flor H. Using interactive immersive VR/AR for the therapy of phantom limb pain. In: Proceedings of the 13th International Conference on Humans and Computers. Aizu-Wakamatsu: University of Aizu Press; 2010.

120. Ortiz-Catalan M, Sander N, Kristoffersen MB, Håkansson B, Brånemark R. Treatment of phantom limb pain (PLP) based on augmented reality and gaming controlled by myoelectric pattern recognition: a case study of a chronic PLP patient. Front Neurosci. 2014;8:24.

121. Lee C, Kim Y, Lee B. Augmented reality-based postural control training improves gait function in patients with stroke: randomized controlled trial. Hong Kong Physiother J. 2014;32(2):51–7.

122. Voss C, Washington P, Haber N, Kline A, Daniels J, Fazel A, De T, McCarthy B, Feinstein C, Winograd T, Wall D. Superpower glass: delivering unobtrusive real-time social cues in wearable systems. In: Proceedings of the 2016 ACM International Joint Conference on Pervasive and Ubiquitous Computing: Adjunct. New York, NY: ACM; 2016.

123. Juan MC, Alcaniz M, Monserrat C, Botella C, Baños RM, Guerrero B. Using augmented reality to treat phobias. IEEE Comput Graph Appl. 2005;25(6):31–7.

124. Botella CM, Juan MC, Baños RM, Alcañiz M, Guillén V, Rey B. Mixing realities? An application of augmented reality for the treatment of cockroach phobia. CyberPsychol Behav. 2005;8(2):162–71.

125. Juan MC, Baños R, Botella C, Pérez D, Alcañiz M, Monserrat C. An augmented reality system for the treatment of acrophobia: the sense of presence using immersive photography. Presence Teleop Virt. 2006;15(4):393–402.

126. Juan MC, Pérez D. Using augmented and virtual reality for the development of acrophobic scenarios. Comparison of the levels of presence and anxiety. Comput Graph. 2010;34(6):756–66.

127. Yeh S, Li Y, Zhou C, Chiu P, Chen J. Effects of virtual reality and augmented reality on induced anxiety. IEEE Trans Neur Syst Rehabil Eng. 2018;26(7):1345–52.

128. Wrzesien M, Burkhardt J, Alcañiz Raya M, Botella C. Mixing psychology and HCI in evaluation of augmented reality mental health technology. In: CHI'11 Extended Abstracts on Human Factors in Computing Systems. New York, NY: ACM; 2011. p. 2119–24.
129. Wrzesien M, et al. How technology influences the therapeutic process: a comparative field evaluation of augmented reality and in vivo exposure therapy for phobia of small animals. In: IFIP Conference on Human-Computer Interaction. New York, NY: Springer; 2011.
130. Wrzesien M, Alcañiz M, Botella C, Burkhardt J, Bretón-López J, Ortega M, et al. The therapeutic lamp: treating small-animal phobias. IEEE Comput Graph Appl. 2013;33(1):80–6.

Using Internet of Things in Healthcare

Riitta Mieronkoski and Sanna Salanterä

Introduction

The Internet of Things (IoT) is a network of interconnected systems that can be controlled remotely over the Internet. The system of multiple devices collects and exchanges data to be analyzed and used for monitoring, maintenance, and process improvements in many industries. In IoT technology the connected things or objects with unique identities are able to interact and cooperate with each other to enable modern wireless telecommunications. The main goal of IoT is to make a computer sense information without or with minimum aid of human intervention to provide customized services [1, 2]. As the IoT technology is mainly invisible and embedded in the environment, it blends seamlessly around us. IoT has already taken over many industries with intelligent solutions: smart cities use IoT to measure air quality and to control the streetlights automatically. Smart transportation solutions tell the citizens for how long they have to wait for the bus, and smart buildings control their energy consumption. However, in healthcare, the concept of IoT is still in its infancy [3, 4].

The use of Radio Frequency IDentification (RFID) to track, monitor, or identify any object and people with tags and wireless connection to the reader has been seen as early applications for IoT [5]. Today, the IoT systems include wireless sensor networks, ubiquitous computation, and various machine learning methods. In 2008 the number of devices "things" connected to the Internet exceeded the number of

R. Mieronkoski (✉)
Department of Nursing Science, University of Turku, Turku, Finland
e-mail: ritemi@utu.fi

S. Salanterä
Department of Nursing Science, University of Turku, Turku, Finland

Turku University Hospital, Turku, Finland
e-mail: sansala@utu.fi

© Springer Nature Switzerland AG 2020
A. Charalambous (ed.), *Developing and Utilizing Digital Technology in Healthcare for Assessment and Monitoring*,
https://doi.org/10.1007/978-3-030-60697-8_8

people being connected to the Internet [6]. This has been seen as a beginning of the IoT even if the term was used already in the end of 1990s [7]. It is estimated that by 2020, the number of devices connected to the Internet will be 50 billion [8].

The main aim of the IoT technology in healthcare is to enable continuous, real-time, automated health monitoring of healthcare customers in different environments. The automatization of the process is expected to increase patient safety and to reduce healthcare costs. The fast development of technology has been seen as a solution for the changes in society with aging population and growing prevalence of chronic deceases.

At the moment, the healthcare system produces a great amount of data, but the collected data have not been used to their fullest potential. The future IoT methods and technologies will enable the data being used for developing the proactiveness and personalization of healthcare. With this, organizations aim to produce more effective and safe health services and high-quality patient-centered care with lower overall costs.

Key Components of IoT

The development of wearable sensor nodes has been one of the key aspects in the IoT in healthcare. Today, the wearables are available in many forms and can be integrated into textile fibers, elastic bands, or directly attached to the human body. The wireless wearable sensors are noninvasive, unobtrusive, and comfortable for the user [9]. Nonintrusive and comfort solution would be a node integrating the needed sensors into portable multipurpose devices [4]. Also, vision-based sensors are used commonly for monitoring patient's physiological parameters and their behavior-related activities [10]. According to a recent market analysis of wearable fitness tracker, wearables for hands are still dominating the customer markets even if other options are already available [11].

The IoT-enabled architectures can be viewed as a four-layer organizational structure, including layers for sensing, networking, data processing, and application [12]. The sensing layer consists of the sensors monitoring the health of patients, actions of the healthcare workers, and the environment. This is the layer closest to the clinical environment of the healthcare and it includes also the medical devices connected to the IoT system. The second layer, networking, connects the sensors to the server through a smart gateway. The gateway transfers the data from the sensing layer using wireless connectivity with, for example, a WiFi or a Bluetooth system. From the gateway the data is transferred to the third layer for data processing. The data analytics and sematic processes take place in the remote cloud server, to obtain knowledge from the heterogeneous data. In the final layer, the application layer, the real-time or off-line processed data is displayed to the end user in monitors in a use-able form. With the "wisdom" processed from the collected data, this can be of direct help to the healthcare personnel for decision making with automatic alarms, notifications, and reminders. Concerning the big data being processed into useful

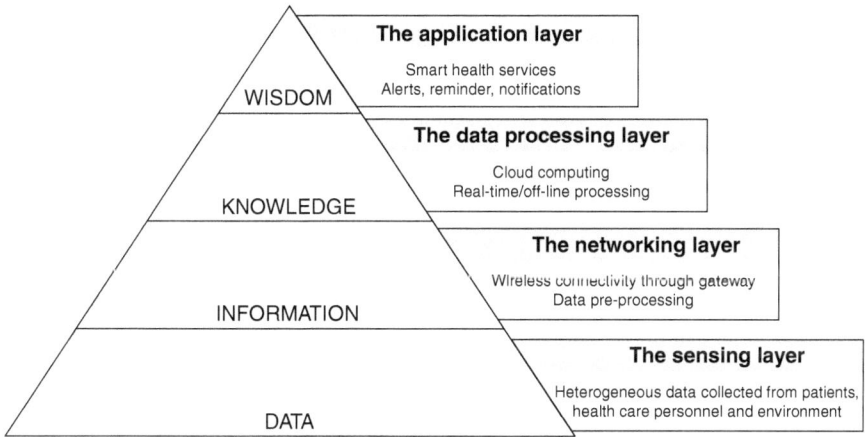

Fig. 1 The process from data to wisdom and the layers of the Internet of Things architecture

form for the smart healthcare services, these layers are viewed parallel to the framework of Data-Information-Knowledge-Wisdom pyramid [13, 14] (Fig. 1).

In healthcare, the technology used involves usually humans—patients or healthcare personnel—which is a challenge because of the complexity of the spectrum of human life. On the contrary, many other industries, also the IoT systems in healthcare, have "human-in-the-loop," which makes the development and the control of the system more complicated. Stankovic [15] describes the human-in-the-loop applications in four types depending of the amount of human involvement in the process: applications controlled by humans, applications where the system passively monitors humans and takes appropriate actions, applications where physiological parameters of the human are modeled, and hybrids of all these types.

Current Literature on IoT

IoT in Hospital Environment

Continuous remote health monitoring with automated data handling is a desired feature to replace the periodic health monitoring done by nurses in the hospital environment. According to a scoping review [3] exploring the literature on IoT used in the technology directed to basic nursing care in a hospital environment, the innovations were targeted to several aspects of patient care. However, the main body of the literature was publised in technological conference proceedings and showed that research on the topic was still in its early stages. There was still a lack of evidence of any implemented IoT technology in basic nursing care to show results in improved care quality or patient safety [3].

In the hospital environment, vital sign monitoring has been the most common area for the IoT innovations. With IoT technology, the vital sign detection methods are versatile and have shown novel solutions for blood pressure, heart rate, breathing rate, and body temperature measurements. For example, respiratory rate can be detected with a small airflow-humidity sensor attached to the nasal prongs or with a paper-based moisture sensor attached to a breathing mask [16, 17]. Many of the innovations aim to be also patient-friendly with more comfortable noninvasive and wearable sensors. For example, a cuffless solution detecting the blood pressure from the pulse wave transit time has been introduced to overcome the challenges in the invasive procedure of continues blood pressure monitoring [18]. The same IoT-based device is also a good example of multi-sensor platforms that detect several vital signs simultaneously [14]; in addition to blood pressure, there is a possibility to monitor real-time heart rate, respiration, temperature, oxygen saturation, and motion of the patient.

The remote monitoring of vital signs in surgical wards has been suggested to decrease the numbers of complications and to reduce the need of activations of the acute response team [19]. Many of the reviewed application for continuous remote monitoring systems had wireless connections and had the ability to communicate with hospital electronic health records (EHR). The potential benefit of automated notifications of the early warning signs of complications has been already studied, but evidence is still lacking [19].

In addition to easily accessible vital signs, also multidimensional and more complicated areas of nursing care have been of interest to the developers of IoT-enabled innovations. A system to monitor incontinence in hospitalized patients includes disposable wetness sensors that can be attached to the diaper. Through wireless connection, the data is transmitted to the cloud and further to the nurses as automated notifications that the diaper is wet. The same kind of wetness detecting biosensors could be used for the detection of wound secretion when attached to a bandage [20]. Also, IoT applications to monitor hand hygiene compliance have been introduced. For example, Baslyman et al. [21] tested a design that integrates an intelligent dispenser with real-time location system. The system is able to detect whether the dispenser is used and sends automated notifications to the healthcare personnel in case the hand hygiene procedures are missed.

IoT in Remote Health Services

The main aim of remote health services is to allow people with health conditions to stay at home instead of being admitted to hospitals or other care facilities. The data from activities (e.g., sleeping and exercise), physiological parameters (e.g., heart rate, body temperature, and breathing rate), symptoms (e.g., pain), or specific health conditions (e.g., diabetes, chronic obstructive pulmonary disease) can be detected real time from a distance. In addition, real-time monitoring of health status could be used for strengthening the patients' engagement for self-care and to empower their healthy lifestyle habits through feedback directly from their portable devices and from their contacts in the healthcare with access to their up-to-date health data.

Flexible and small sensor nodes can be attached to many materials, and wearable devices from smart rings and watches to textiles are already available on the market for a reasonable price. However, it is notable that devices targeted for fitness tracking may not be applicable to be used in healthcare for detecting health conditions without comprehensive evaluation and testing. Also, there might be challenges in implementing these devices into health monitoring systems in healthcare institutions [4].

Remote health monitoring with IoT systems is already tested in many facilities both for the treatment and prevention of health conditions as well as for symptom management. For example, a system with body-worn sensors aiming at monitoring diseases severity by predicting the potential disease has been tested in student healthcare [22]. A recent review by Basatheh et al. [23] found that IoT technology could be used in diabetic foot care for supporting patients with chronic foot ulcers and other foot-related complications in home care. The user acceptance and the feasibility of a commercial wristband have been evaluated to monitor the activities of daily living in mothers in maternal care [24]. Also, IoT-enabling systems have also been proposed in many application for pain assessment and management; however, the development is still in an early stage and the applications suffer from security and privacy problems [25].

IoT in Older Adult Care

Older adult care in home environment is one of the main areas where the IoT-enabled technology could be used. Smart living environments support the elderly to live at home comfortably and independently in a safe environment with ubiquitous monitoring. The automated processes of IoT technology can cover tasks with minimum human interventions and ease the burden of the formal and informal care givers. In the future, IoT technology could offer fully personalized processes to the elderly living at home but with needs for health services. These tasks can be related to the automatization of the living environment including the remote control and maintenance of the devices and systems in the house or related to the monitoring of the health of the resident. However, research related to smart home technology shows that evidence to support aging in place in people with complex health problems is still low and the readiness level of the technology is in an early stage [26].

The potential possibilities of multifunctional wearable sensing materials in the care of the aged has been reviewed by Armstrong et al. [27]. They suggest that when combined with the newer generation of wearable and implantable technologies, significant synergies may emerge in geriatric care environment. When the context is home, where people spend a lot of their time, the passive monitoring of continuous, longitudinal, and multimodal data of individuals and their relation is possible [28].

One of the main areas in smart home monitoring for older adult care is fall detection and fall prevention. Various methods have been tested, including wrist worn accelerometer sensors [29] and vision-based methods with multi-camera systems, monocular systems, and bio-inspired stereo vision [10].

One of the major challenges in smart home technology is data security and privacy issues, and a recent literature has also concentrated on dealing with proposing solutions for these [30]. Also, Baig et al. [31] raise an important and often neglected question about the state of the end user acceptability and usability of the application in recent research concerning the IoT technology targeted for older adult care. They suggest that the usability and acceptability issues could be addressed by early engagement with stakeholders, end users, and clinicians, with a deeper understanding of the current problem the technology is addressed to and with successful co-designs [31].

Current Challenges and Estimated Benefits

There are relatively few direct disadvantages to using IoT technology to serve the needs of healthcare and patients. However, for successful implementation, the risks in information security and privacy must be assessed from multiple angles. In addition, transparency of the processes, consent to use the data, data sharing, and data ownership are major challenges. Energy consumption is one of the technological challenges that is constantly improving.

In IoT technology, the data security risk can be observed one layer at a time. One of the challenges using wearables sensors in remote monitoring is that the healthcare customers in remote monitoring must wear the sensors according to the manufacturer's advice. The accuracy of the data collected in wearable sensors depends on the quality of the signals collected. If the data is disturbed by a variety of noises, caused by poor electrode contact, wrong sensor placement, and motion artifacts, also the final results will be unreliable. Therefore, a continuous support should be available for users in remote health monitoring. The development of sensor calibration techniques and reliable connectivity protocols has been seen as necessary to minimize missing data, which could result in wrong conclusions [15]. Also, there is risk with the data associated with the latency of the real-time data and high energy consumption that should be addressed [32]. One of the key data security risks is users themselves with either unintentional or malicious behavior. The data with personal information can be leaked, contaminated, or lost. It should be carefully considered, who can get access to the data.

In the comprehensive report by the Open Effect [33] reviewing the commercial fitness trackers for security and privacy, the authors found that most of them had security vulnerabilities and the policies of data ownership were unclear. However, data sharing is necessary to enable long-term learning. The concerns of privacy and security can eventually have an impact also on the growth of the market of fitness tracker devices targeted to the customers [11].

The benefits of IoT technology is not limited to the clinical work in healthcare. The use of IoT applications is a promising way to collect continuous data in research as well as creating new knowledge about the phenomena of human life. Cox et al. [34] suggest that passive sensing data could be used for clinical trials in cancer care. Examples of these would be behavioral changes and changes in activity level, heart rate, and sleep patterns of the research participants. In the development process of technologies to automatically detect multidimensional complex symptoms such as pain, new knowledge has been created concerning the behavior. One example is the study by Werner at al. [35] which detected facial pain expression and head pose during painful event.

Baig et al. [31] raise an important issue about the advantages of the IoT technology to support patient's self-engagement. The opportunity for rich interaction between the patient and the healthcare personnel through the technology could be more emphasized instead of seeing the technology merely in a way to collect data. The user perspective of the human-in-the-loop in IoT technology could be more highlighted in the development process. Nurses, who work in close contact with patients and use various devices daily in their work, should be included more strongly in the development.

The role of nursing in the development IoT-enabled technology has not been described in scientific literature. However, Matinolli et al. [36] have explored the role of nurses in the development of health and medical devices directed for fundamental nursing care. The review process revealed that only few research articles described the development process in detail. Out of 19 originally selected papers describing the developed devices, the role of nurses could only be identified in five studies. The development process was mainly described in three phases: defining the need, prototyping, and testing. While defining the need, the researchers conducted field studies, including questionnaires and interviews of requirement and expectations for the new device. The prototyping phase was reported only as a technical process and no description of nurse involvement could be identified. In testing and implementing phases, the devices were tested in clinical settings and testing included patients in addition to healthy volunteers. Also, nurses' viewpoints were studied in some cases to ensure the usability [36]. There is a definite need to have nurses better involved in this kind of research in order to better meet the needs of nurses.

Conclusions

There is a need for low-cost and easy-to-use solutions to monitor health-related factors in the present and future healthcare. IoT-enabled solutions are bringing new strategies to provide personalized and proactive healthcare services. Bringing the IoT to its full potential in healthcare demands high interdisciplinary skills. Successful development and implementation should involve specialists from multiple disciplines and applied areas such as engineering, computer science, information technology, medicine, nursing, and social sciences. Nurses, as one of the key actors in healthcare, have mainly a positive attitude to technology. However, nurses are still rarely included in the process of device development. Engineers, healthcare workers, and researchers should work in synergy to advance the implementation of IoT in healthcare and to face major challenges of the new paradigm in the complex and sensitive environment.

The future research should be focused on the implementation and effectiveness of the technology in healthcare and the involvement of the end users in the development process to ensure the user-centric design. The use of commercial applications of smart devices in healthcare should be taken with caution due to multiple data security and privacy challenges. Along with security challenges, also ethical issues should be considered in the development of smart systems for the use of various facilities in healthcare.

References

1. Gubbi J, Buyya R, Marusic S, Palaniswami M. Internet of Things (IoT): a vision, architectural elements, and future directions. Futur Gener Comput Syst. 2013;29(7):1645–60.
2. Atzori L, Iera A, Morabito G. The internet of things: a survey. Comput Netw. 2010;54:2787–805.
3. Mieronkoski R, Azimi I, Rahmani AM, Aantaa R, Terävä V, Liljeberg P, et al. The Internet of Things for basic nursing care—a scoping review. Int J Nurs Stud. 2017;69:78–90.
4. Baker SB, Xiang W, Atkinson I. Internet of things for smart healthcare: technologies, challenges, and opportunities. IEEE Access. 2017;5:26521–44.
5. Jia X, Feng Q, Fan T, Lei Q. RFID technology and its applications in Internet of Things (IoT). In: 2012 2nd International Conference on Consumer Electronics, Communications and Networks, CECNet 2012 - Proceedings; 2012. p. 1282–5.
6. Cisco. How the next evolution of the internet is changing everything. White paper. CISCO White Pap. 2011;1:1–11.
7. Oriwoh E, Conrad M. "Things" in the internet of things: towards a definition. Int J Internet Things. 2015;4(1):1–5.
8. Anderson J, Rainie L. The future of smart systems. Pew Research Center. 2012. https://www.pewresearch.org/internet/2012/06/29/the-future-of-smart-systems/#fn-163-1.
9. Majumder S, Mondal T, Deen MJ. Wearable sensors for remote health monitoring. Sensors. 2017;17:130.
10. Sathyanarayana S, Satzoda RK, Sathyanarayana S, Thambipillai S. Vision-based patient monitoring: a comprehensive review of algorithms and technologies. J Ambient Intell Humaniz Comput. 2018;9(2):225–51.
11. Market data forecast. Fitness trackers market share, size & growth. 2019 - 2025. https://www.marketdataforecast.com/market-reports/fitness-trackers-market.
12. Da Xu L, He W, Li S. Internet of things in industries: a survey. IEEE Trans Ind Informatics. 2014;10:2233–43.
13. Thomson R, Lebiere C, Bennati S. Human, model and machine: a complementary approach to big data. ACM Int Conf Proc Ser. 2014:27–31.
14. Swan M. Sensor mania! The internet of things, wearable computing, objective metrics, and the quantified self 2.0. J Sens Actuator Netw. 2012;1(3):217–53.
15. Stankovic JA. Research directions for the internet of things. IEEE Internet Things J. 2014;1(1):3–9.

16. André N, Druart S, Gérard P, Pampin R, Moreno-Hagelsieb L, Kezai T, et al. Miniaturized wireless sensing system for real-time breath activity recording. IEEE Sensors J. 2010;10(1):178–84.

17. Güder F, Ainla A, Redston J, Mosadegh B, Glavan A, Martin TJ, et al. Paper-based electrical respiration sensor. Angew Chem Int Ed. 2016;55(19):5727–32.

18. Fang Z, Zhao Z, Sun F, Chen X, Du L, Li H, et al. The 3AHcare node: health monitoring continuously. In: 2012 IEEE 14th International Conference on e-Health Networking, Applications and Services, Healthcom 2012. Washington, DC: IEEE; 2012. p. 365–6.

19. Boer C, Touw HR, Loer SA. Postanesthesia care by remote monitoring of vital signs in surgical wards. Curr Opin Anaesthesiol. 2018;31:716–22.

20. Fuketa H, Yoshioka K, Yokota T, Yukita W, Koizumi M, Sekino M, et al. Organic-transistor-based 2kV ESD-tolerant flexible wet sensor sheet for biomedical applications with wireless power and data transmission using 13.56MHz magnetic resonance. In: Digest of Technical Papers - IEEE International Solid-State Circuits Conference. Washington, DC: IEEE; 2014. p. 490–1.

21. Baslyman M, Rezaee R, Amyot D, Mouttham A, Chreyh R, Geiger G, et al. Real-time and location-based hand hygiene monitoring and notification: proof-of-concept system and experimentation. Pers Ubiquit Comput. 2015;19(3):667–88.

22. Verma P, Sood SK, Kalra S. Cloud-centric IoT based student healthcare monitoring framework. J Ambient Intell Humaniz Comput. 2018;9(5):1293–309.

23. Basatneh R, Najafi B, Armstrong DG. Health sensors, smart home devices, and the internet of medical things: an opportunity for dramatic improvement in care for the lower extremity complications of diabetes. J Diabetes Sci Technol. 2018;12(3):577–86.

24. Grym K, Niela-Vilén H, Ekholm E, Hamari L, Azimi I, Rahmani A, et al. Feasibility of smart wristbands for continuous monitoring during pregnancy and one month after birth. BMC Pregn Childb. 2019;19(1):34.

25. Argüello Prada EJ. The Internet of Things (IoT) in pain assessment and management: an overview. Informatics Med Unlocked. 2020;18:100298.

26. Liu L, Stroulia E, Nikolaidis I, Miguel-Cruz A, Rios RA. Smart homes and home health monitoring technologies for older adults: a systematic review. Int J Med Inform. 2016;91:44–59.

27. Armstrong DG, Najafi B, Shahinpoor M. Potential applications of smart multifunctional wearable materials to gerontology. Gerontology. 2017;63(3):287–98.

28. Nelson BW, Allen NB. Extending the passive-sensing toolbox: using smart-home technology in psychological science. Perspect Psychol Sci. 2018;13(6):718–33.

29. Khojasteh S, Villar J, Chira C, González V, de la Cal E. Improving fall detection using an on-wrist wearable accelerometer. Sensors. 2018;18(5):1350.

30. Alkhatib S, Waycott J, Buchanan G, Bosua R. Privacy and the internet of things (IoT) monitoring solutions for older adults: a review. Stud Health Technol Inform. 2018;252:8–14.

31. Baig MM, Afifi S, GholamHosseini H, Mirza F. A Systematic review of wearable sensors and IoT-based monitoring applications for older adults – a focus on ageing population and independent living. J Med Syst. 2019;43:233.

32. Rault T, Bouabdallah A, Challal Y, Marin F. A survey of energy-efficient context recognition systems using wearable sensors for healthcare applications. Pervas Mob Comput. 2017;37:23. https://hal.archives-ouvertes.fr/hal-01466848.

33. Hilts A, Parsons C, Knockel J. Every step you fake: a comparative analysis of fitness tracker privacy and security. 2016. https://openeffect.ca/reports/Every_Step_You_Fake.pdf.

34. Cox SM, Lane A, Volchenboum SL. Use of wearable, mobile, and sensor technology in cancer clinical trials. JCO Clin Cancer Informatics. 2018;2:1–11.

35. Werner P, Al-Hamadi A, Niese R, Walter S, Gruss S, Traue H. Towards pain monitoring: facial expression, head pose, a new database, an automatic system and remaining challenges. 2014.

36. Matinolli HM, Mieronkoski R, Salanterä S. Health and medical device development for fundamental care: scoping review. J Clin Nurs. 2020;29:1822.

The Use of Gaming in Healthcare

Anni Pakarinen and Sanna Salanterä

Introduction

Key Concepts

Multiple definitions exists on games, health games, and gamification. Next, we offer the definitions of these key concepts according to few key sources.

Game Game is a system that involves different components, such as players, rules, goals, competition, and opponents [1–4]. Traditionally games have been used for fun and entertainment, but *serious games* are a genre of games that are used for other purposes than simply for entertainment [1, 5, 6]. Serious games can be considered as an umbrella concept for different types of serious games that are used for various purposes like for education, military, government, corporate, and healthcare [6].

Health games Health games are serious games that are developed and/or used for different kinds of health-related purposes. Entertaining games, such as commercially available active games, can be called as health games as well, if they are used for health-related purposes, e.g., in rehabilitation. Moreover, educational games can

A. Pakarinen (✉)
Department of Nursing Science, University of Turku, Turku, Finland
e-mail: anni.pakarinen@utu.fi

S. Salanterä
Department of Nursing Science, University of Turku, Turku, Finland

Turku University Hospital, Turku, Finland
e-mail: sansala@utu.fi

© Springer Nature Switzerland AG 2020   115
A. Charalambous (ed.), *Developing and Utilizing Digital Technology in Healthcare for Assessment and Monitoring*,
https://doi.org/10.1007/978-3-030-60697-8_9

be health games, if they aim to educate patients, clients, and professionals on health-related issues [7–9].

Gamification Gamification means the use of game elements in nongame contexts [10]. The purpose is to use the elements from games that make them interesting and attractive [11, 12]. Gamification is nowadays a rapidly growing trend in many areas [12], also in healthcare. According to a recent review on gamification supporting mental health and well-being, the most used gamification elements were levels or feedback for progress, scoring or points, prizes or rewards, theme or narrative, customization, and personalization [13].

Different Types of Health Games

There are multiple ways to distribute games into different categories. Next, we offer definitions of game types following several distribution approaches. The list is not exhaustive and mutually exclusive, but highlights typical types of games also used for health-related purposes. Games are distributed according to the device used or platform, like *mobile games*, computer or *PC games,* and *console games.* Further, games may be divided according to the way gaming occurs, like *active games* or *exergames*, where the movements of the player are used to control the game as opposed to *sedentary games*, where the control of the game is based on the game controller or keyboard and mouse [14]. Simulation and virtual reality are also broadly used approaches in health games. In *simulation games*, the game elements are copying various activities from real world [15] and in *virtual reality (VR) games*, a three-dimensional artificial environment that uses realistic images, videos, sounds, and other sensations offers gamers a simulation of physical presence in a virtual environment [16]. Further, in *augmented reality (AR) games*, perspective of real physical environment and computer-generated imagery are synthesized, often in real time and three dimensionally [17]. The VR and AR technologies have led to *pervasive games*, in which real-world games are synthesized with computer-generated functionality [18].

Multiple distributions have been proposed for health games also in previous research publications. Baranowski et al. [8] divided health games according to the intended outcome expectation of the game: (1) games that increase health-relevant knowledge, (2) games that change health-related behavior, (3) games that involve health-related behavior change in game play, and (4) games that influence health precursors. In their review, Kharrazi et al. [19] divided games according to the intended purpose: (1) rehab games for rehabilitation, (2) exercise games to support physical exercise, (3) behavioral games to affect player's behavior (e.g., medication adherence), (4) educational games to inform player's about different health issues, (5) cognitive games to support cognitive performance, and (6) hybrid games, which are a mix of others.

The Advantages and Challenges of Gaming in Healthcare

The Advantages of Games

Several game-based mechanics are built on the idea of the engagement, enjoyment, and motivation of gamers, which make games also one potential method for health promotion [20]. Because of the fun and attractive nature of games, they are played regardless of age, gender, and background [21]. Games enable reaching the patients and clients no matter the time and distance. They also enable collecting and storing different types of health data on individuals [8, 22]. Many of the games are also readily accessible and easy to use, because they are built on platforms that are already familiar to users. Research shows that health games help reach those that are difficult to reach with traditional health promotion methods [8, 23].

Games can be used to practice different skills, and thus are used to train and educate healthcare personnel or students, for example in practicing patient care, manual skills, and decision-making. Games enable practicing skills that are impossible to practice otherwise in real-life environments. Different scenarios may be offered through games more easily than in real-life settings, because of cost, time, and ethical restraints [24]. Games may also be used to train and educate patients and clients, for example about health habits, preparation for operation, and about diseases or medication [14]. The health content may also be embedded into the game design such that gamers are discretely exposed to it only by playing [20, 25].

Sensibly developed games encourage setting and reaching health-related goals. Games can support interactive learning and communication. They enable to establish peer-support groups and communication between the professional and patient or client, for example to give feedback on progress in rehabilitation. Games may foster patient-centered care. They enable tailored content and feedback according to the individual needs of the users. Games may be developed for healthy people and people with different health conditions, disabilities, and risk factors, as well as for different age groups [14, 26, 27].

Among children and youth, games have showed positive results as regards health outcomes. Active games increased energy expenditure among healthy adolescents [28] and improved Body Mass Index (BMI) among overweight and obese children [29]. Active games improved motor skills among healthy pre-school aged children [30] and among children with movement disorders [31, 32]. Active games also improved balance among children and adolescents with lower limb amputation [33] and children with movement disorders [32]. Virtual reality game alleviated pain during painful procedures, specially the process of changing bandages, among children with acute burn injuries [34]. In addition to physical outcomes, different positive outcomes on mental and psychological health are evidenced. Cognitive Behavior Therapy-based games and gamification had positive effects on mental health, like reduction in depressive symptoms and anxiety among children and youth [35]. Videogames and mobile health applications were found feasible delivering empowerment interventions to pediatric cancer patients [36].

Many game-based studies have explored the effects of games from the perspective of knowledge and behavior [14]. Educational games improved nutritional knowledge among healthy children [37] and among overweight and obese children [38]. Games also increased knowledge among children with asthma [39, 40] and young people with diabetes and cancer [39]. In addition to increased knowledge, games may support adherence to medication or other treatment [14]. Educational games improved self-management in young people with asthma, diabetes, and cancer [39] and gamification and virtual games provided positive reinforcement, increased extrinsic motivation, and self-management among children with diabetes [41]. Active games increased light-to-moderate physical activity among healthy children and youth [42, 43] and among overweight and obese children [38]. Serious games and gamification increased fruit and vegetable intake among children [37]. Games are also potential in promoting psychological determinants for behavior change, like physical activity self-efficacy [44].

Even the research among children and youth is more prevalent, there are also positive findings of games among adults [45] and elderly [46]. Active games showed their promise in improvement of health and wellness of older adults [47] and had potentially positive results for depressive symptoms [35]. Active games also increased physical activity in the short term among adults [48] and energy expenditure among post-stroke patients and among people with mild severity cerebral palsy [49]. Virtual reality games improved mobility and balance among elderly [50] and provided positive reinforcement, increased extrinsic motivation, and self-management among adults and elderly with diabetes [41]. Virtual Reality (VR) and Augmented Reality (AR) had also positive results for different mental health outcomes [35]. Gamification had positive impact on different health behaviors [51] and provided positive reinforcement, increased extrinsic motivation, and self-management among adults and elderly with diabetes [41].

Challenges of Games

With the knowledge of the advantages of games, there are also several challenges to be considered from the perspective of gaming in healthcare. Firstly, from the users' perspective, healthcare professionals' knowledge, skills, and attitudes are issues that affect the implementation process of games in healthcare. It should be considered what kind of training and change management actions are needed before new technologies are fluently rooted in healthcare practices [52]. Same issues are important also from the perspective of patients and clients to ensure the equal accessibility of games. Everyone in the target group should have the same possibility to play the health game and understand the content [52–54].

Second, from the perspective of the organization, practical issues in everyday work may occur, like how to take care of infection risks of different games and their hardware. When acquiring health technology, healthcare providers have to think about the issues of costs, maintenance, and updates, but also the security and safety issues. Questions usually arise, when something unaccepted happens, for example, who holds the responsibility in the case of accidents during gameplay or health data leakages [52, 53, 55]. In addition, health games are usually not regarded as medical devices, leading to uncertainty of their quality and validity to be implemented in healthcare. Even though there are some frameworks and tools trying to tackle this challenge [52], there are no commonly approved certification system or quality appraisal tools for health games [52, 53, 56].

Certain issues in gaming are critical, especially among children and adolescents. Gaming may lead to negative physical and mental health problems. The immersive nature of games may lead to excessive gaming. This may influence physical health through increased inactivity and sedentary behavior [57, 58]. Excessive gaming may lead also to sleeping difficulties, behavioral problems, and learning difficulties at school [59, 60]. A small proportion of gamers suffer from game addiction, which may lead to problems in social life and producing social exclusion of individuals [60, 61]. These should be regarded also when adult gamers are concerned, but there is limited research on gaming among adult populations from this perspective [61].

All of these challenges should be considered already from the beginning of the development process of health games to tackle the challenges and to end up with credible, valuable, and valid game-based methods to be implemented in healthcare [52, 53].

Development and Evaluation of Games

Development Through User-Centered Design Process

Effective health games are end products of a rigorous process, designed based on theory and evidence, developed and tested among target group, and evaluated thoroughly in laboratory settings, intended contexts, and among target group [62]. Absence of thorough design, development, and evaluation of the health game may end up with resentment of users, low efficiency, increased costs, interference of workflow, and increase in errors in care [63–66]. User-centeredness in game design and development is a method and a process where the demands and insight of the target group are given substantial attention at every step. The development process is iterative and calls for multi-professional team that consists of different skills and views [63, 65–67]. Sustainable implementation of the different components of the game also call for user-centered design principles [68, 69].

Below we present a step-by-step framework for development and evaluation of health games (Picture 1), following user-centered design principles. These principles aim at achievement of immersion, sustained attention, and engagement among users, as well as promotion of understanding on health matters embedded in the game [7, 70]. These principles include multi-professional capacity in the development team, needs assessment, and insight of the users throughout the development process [8, 63].

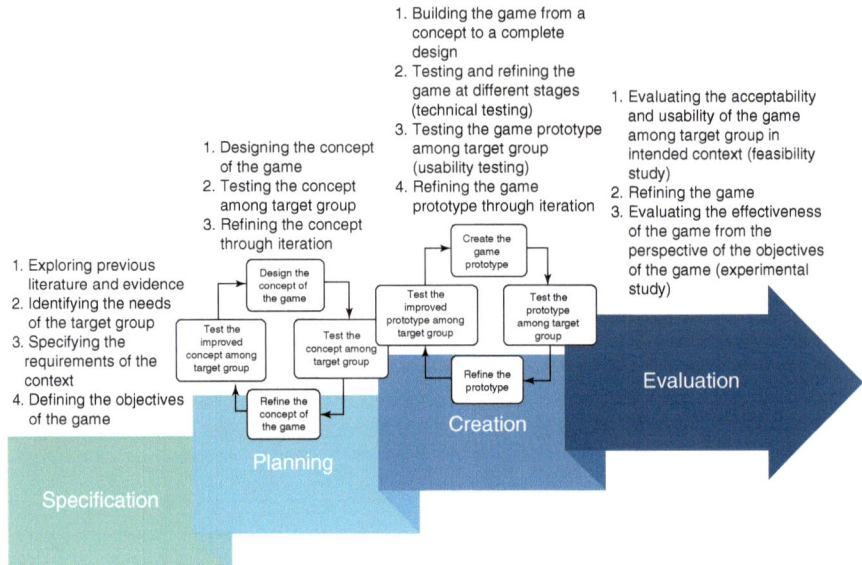

Picture 1 A step-by-step framework for development and evaluation of health games

Specification A multi-professional development team, consisting of experts in the content of health and behavioral sciences as well as experts in hardware and software development, visualization, and graphics design [8, 71], aims at ensuring the validity of the content from the perspective of health, as well as improving the game content and the system. This phase includes identification and analysis of previous knowledge and theory related to the health topic. Questions to be asked at this phase may include the following: What is the current situation related to the health topic? What needs to be changed, learned, or promoted? Is there any guiding theory related to the health topic and intervention objectives? Are the objectives possible to achieve with game? Are there any previous games related to the health topic? Which are the game elements with promising effects? After the identification and analyses of evidence and theory, the needs, views, and perceptions of the target group related to the health topic and game content should be assessed [63, 66, 69], for example by conducting empirical studies among them. The profound understanding of the target group guides defining the objectives for the game. This phase also includes specifying the requirements of the context of use [63, 66, 69] by identifying the persons who will use the game, what they will use it for, and under what conditions they will use it.

Planning First phase in game development guides the designing of the concept for the game by setting the basis for the game. It guides the design of the content of the game, the game elements, mechanics, and health content, but may also help to construct a theory-based framework for the game. Studies among users support also the content design, and choosing relevant devices, platforms, and software. Besides the game design, first phase also guides the planning of need-based training materials for the end users. Users are also involved at this phase, since their perceptions from the perspective of the game concept are valuable before proceeding to the actual creation of the game. Concept testing is usually an iterative process, where the concept and mock-ups are refined in between the user testing.

Creation The actual development of the game is usually done through several stages of iteration. The game is created from rough first version to the final prototype and technical stability, quality, and usability of the game are tested between iterations (alpha, beta) [72]. These formative tests are usually small-scale studies aiming to detect and fix problems in game technicalities. After the prototype is ready, the usability of the game is tested among targeted end users. Usability tests enable testing the ease of use, functionality, usefulness, understandability, relevance, and visualization of the game [63, 66].

Evaluation of Games Before Implementation in Healthcare

Evaluation Before implementing new interventions, their feasibility should be evaluated. Optimally the feasibility of health games is evaluated in intended contexts. Thus, feasibility studies are usually conducted in real-life contexts, like hospitals, and among intended end users. Feasibility studies show whether health game is appropriate and relevant for implementation, and what kind of modifications and changes are needed. Feasibility studies enable various issues to be evaluated, like usability, acceptability, and initial effectiveness of the health game, where acceptability refers to the attractiveness, suitability, satisfaction, and perceived appropriateness of the health game among intended end users [68, 73].

Effectivity of the health games should also be tested before the game is implemented. There the interest is in what is needed to reach the expected outcomes with playing the game [73]. This assessment can include several perspectives, e.g., how much time is needed to reach the goal, how cost-effective the game is, what are the needs of the target group, what does it take to master the topic, is it really changing behavior/increasing knowledge/increasing physical activity/improving health outcomes or improving cognitive skills. Descriptive, comparative, quasi-experimental, or experimental study designs as well as economical evaluations can be used. These studies require lengthy data collection periods and follow-up times [19]. Usually the game interventions require a series of studies from testing the theoretical basis, defining the elements of the game, piloting, and actual intervention study.

Conclusion

Games are attractive and engaging and therefore have potential in the field of health and health promotion. Serious games—as all games—are systems that involve components such as players, rules, goals, and competition. Gamification uses game elements in nongame contexts. Health games are of various types that can be played on mobile phones, consoles, and computers. They can be active or sedentary, and simulated, virtual or pervasive. Health games can aim at improving health, increasing knowledge, cognitive skills, change behavior, or influence precursors (e.g., increase health literacy). Games have both advantages and challenges that should be taken into account in designing them. Health games can be designed for different age groups with different health problems, or they can be aimed at anyone. Health games should be developed rigorously in thorough processes and with well-designed studies. Usability, feasibility, and effectiveness evaluation should all be included in the development of health games.

References

1. Adams E. Fundamentals of game design. London: Pearson Education; 2014.
2. Salen K, Tekinbaş KS, Zimmerman E. Rules of play: game design fundamentals. Cambridge: MIT press; 2004.
3. Smed J, Hakonen H. Towards a definition of a computer game. Turku: Turku Centre for Computer Science; 2003.
4. Suits B. What is a game? Philos Sci. 1967;34(2):148–56.
5. Djaouti D, Alvarez J, Jessel J, Rampnoux O. Origins of serious games. In: Serious games and edutainment applications. London: Springer; 2011. p. 25–43.
6. Susi T, Johannesson M, Backlund P (2007) Serious games: an overview
7. Baranowski T, Buday R, Thompson DI, Baranowski J. Playing for real: video games and stories for health-related behavior change. Am J Prev Med. 2008;34(1):74–82.
8. Baranowski T, Blumberg F, Buday R, DeSmet A, Fiellin LE, Green CS, Kato PM, Lu AS, Maloney AE, Mellecker R. Games for health for children—current status and needed research. Games Health J. 2016;5(1):1–2.
9. Lu AS, Baranowski T, Thompson D, Buday R. Story immersion of videogames for youth health promotion: a review of literature. Games Health Res Dev Clin Appl. 2012;1(3):199–204.
10. Deterding S, Khaled R, Nacke LE, Dixon D. Gamification: toward a definition. In: CHI 2011 Gamification Workshop Proceedings 2011, Vancouver BC, Canada, vol. 12.
11. Liu D, Santhanam R, Webster J. Toward meaningful engagement: a framework for design and research of gamified information systems. MIS Q. 2017;41(4):1011.
12. Morschheuser B, Hassan L, Werder K, Hamari J. How to design gamification? A method for engineering gamified software. Inf Softw Technol. 2018;95:219–37.
13. Cheng VW, Davenport T, Johnson D, Vella K, Hickie IB. Gamification in apps and technologies for improving mental health and well-being: systematic review. JMIR Mental Health. 2019;6(6):e13717.
14. Parisod H, Pakarinen A, Kauhanen L, Aromaa M, Leppänen V, Liukkonen TN, Smed J, Salanterä S. Promoting children's health with digital games: a review of reviews. Games Health Res Dev Clin Appl. 2014;3(3):145–56.
15. Jones K. Simulations: a handbook for teachers and trainers. London: Routledge; 2013.

16. Noghabaei M, Asadi K, Han K. Virtual manipulation in an immersive virtual environment: simulation of virtual assembly. In: Proceedings of the Computing in Civil Engineering; 2019.
17. Azuma RT. A survey of augmented reality. Pres Teleoper Virt Environ. 1997;6(4):355–85.
18. Soute I, Markopoulos P, Magielse R. Head Up Games: combining the best of both worlds by merging traditional and digital play. Pers Ubiquit Comput. 2010;14(5):435–44.
19. Kharrazi H, Lu AS, Gharghabi F, Coleman W. A scoping review of health game research: past, present, and future. Games Health Res Dev Clin Appl. 2012;1(2):153–64.
20. Hamari J, Koivisto J, Sarsa H. Does gamification work?--a literature review of empirical studies on gamification. In: 2014 47th Hawaii International Conference on System Sciences. Washington, DC: IEEE; 2014. p. 3025–34.
21. Entertainment Software Association. Essential facts about the computer and video game industry. 2019.
22. Staiano AE, Calvert SL. The promise of exergames as tools to measure physical health. Entertain Comput. 2011;2(1):17–21.
23. DeSmet A, Thompson D, Baranowski T, Palmeira A, Verloigne M, De Bourdeaudhuij I. Is participatory design associated with the effectiveness of serious digital games for healthy lifestyle promotion? A meta-analysis. J Med Internet Res. 2016;18(4):e94.
24. Gentry SV, Gauthier A, Ehrstrom BL, Wortley D, Lilienthal A, Car LT, Dauwels-Okutsu S, Nikolaou CK, Zary N, Campbell J, Car J. Serious gaming and gamification education in health professions: systematic review. J Med Internet Res. 2019;21(3):e12994.
25. Seaborn K, Fels DI. Gamification in theory and action: a survey. Int J Hum Comput Stud. 2015;74:14–31.
26. Laamarti F, Eid M, El Saddik A. An overview of serious games. Int J Comput Games Technol. 2014;2014:358152.
27. Nøhr C, Aarts J. Use of "serious health games" in health care: a review. In: Information Technology in Health Care: Socio-Technical Approaches 2010: from Safe Systems to Patient Safety, vol. 157; 2010. p. 160.
28. Barnett A, Cerin E, Baranowski T. Active video games for youth: a systematic review. J Phys Act Health. 2011;8(5):724–37.
29. Koenig HG. Impact of game-based health promotion programs on body mass index in over-weight/obese children and adolescents: a systematic review and meta-analysis of randomized con-trolled trials. Child Obes. 2018;14:67.
30. Barnett LM, Hinkley T, Okely AD, Hesket K, Salmon JO. Use of electronic games by young children and fundamental movement skills? Percept Mot Skills. 2012;114(3):1023–34.
31. Hickman R, Popescu L, Manzanares R, Morris B, Lee SP, Dufek JS. Use of active video gaming in children with neuromotor dysfunction: a systematic review. Dev Med Child Neurol. 2017;59(9):903–11.
32. Page ZE, Barrington S, Edwards J, Barnett LM. Do active video games benefit the motor skill development of non-typically developing children and adolescents: a systematic review. J Sci Med Sport. 2017;20(12):1087–100.
33. Andrysek J, Klejman S, Steinnagel B, Torres-Moreno R, Zabjek KF, Salbach NM, Moody K. Preliminary evaluation of a commercially available videogame system as an adjunct therapeutic intervention for improving balance among children and adolescents with lower limb amputations. Arch Phys Med Rehabil. 2012;93(2):358–66.
34. Das DA, Grimmer KA, Sparnon AL, McRae SE, Thomas BH. The efficacy of playing a virtual reality game in modulating pain for children with acute burn injuries: a randomized controlled trial [ISRCTN87413556]. BMC Pediatr. 2005;5(1):1.
35. Fleming TM, Bavin L, Stasiak K, Hermansson-Webb E, Merry SN, Cheek C, Lucassen M, Lau HM, Pollmuller B, Hetrick S. Serious games and gamification for mental health: current status and promising directions. Front Psychiatry. 2017;7:215.
36. Govender M, Bowen RC, German ML, Bulaj G, Bruggers CS. Clinical and neurobiological perspectives of empowering pediatric cancer patients using videogames. Games Health J. 2015;4(5):362–74.

37. Chow CY, Riantiningtyas RR, Kanstrup MB, Papavasileiou M, Liem DG, Olsen A. Can games change children's eating behaviour? A review of gamification and serious games. Food Qual Prefer. 2019;80:103823.

38. Guy S, Ratzki-Leewing A, Gwadry-Sridhar F. Moving beyond the stigma: systematic review of video games and their potential to combat obesity. Int J Hypertens. 2011;2011:179124.

39. Charlier N, Zupancic N, Fieuws S, Denhaerynck K, Zaman B, Moons P. Serious games for improving knowledge and self-management in young people with chronic conditions: a systematic review and meta-analysis. J Am Med Inform Assoc. 2016;23(1):230–9.

40. Drummond D, Monnier D, Tesnière A, Hadchouel A. A systematic review of serious games in asthma education. Pediatr Allergy Immunol. 2017;28(3):257–65.

41. Theng YL, Lee JW, Patinadan PV, Foo SS. The use of videogames, gamification, and virtual environments in the self-management of diabetes: a systematic review of evidence. Games Health J. 2015;4(5):352–61.

42. Biddiss E, Irwin J. Active video games to promote physical activity in children and youth: a systematic review. Arch Pediatr Adolesc Med. 2010;164(7):664–72.

43. Peng W, Crouse JC, Lin JH. Using active video games for physical activity promotion: a systematic review of the current state of research. Health Educ Behav. 2013;40(2):171–92.

44. Pakarinen A, Parisod H, Smed J, Salanterä S. Health game interventions to enhance physical activity self-efficacy of children: a quantitative systematic review. J Adv Nurs. 2017;73(4):794–811.

45. Connolly TM, Boyle EA, MacArthur E, Hainey T, Boyle JM. A systematic literature review of empirical evidence on computer games and serious games. Comput Educ. 2012;59(2):661–86.

46. Wiemeyer J, Kliem A. Serious games in prevention and rehabilitation—a new panacea for elderly people? Eur Rev Aging Phys Act. 2012;9(1):41.

47. Kappen DL, Mirza-Babaei P, Nacke LE. Older adults' physical activity and exergames: a systematic review. Int J Hum Comput Interact. 2019;35(2):140–67.

48. Street TD, Lacey SJ, Langdon RR. Gaming your way to health: a systematic review of exergaming programs to increase health and exercise behaviors in adults. Games Health J. 2017;6(3):136–46.

49. Deutsch JE, Guarrera-Bowlby P, Myslinski MJ, Kafri M. Is there evidence that active videogames increase energy expenditure and exercise intensity for people poststroke and with cerebral palsy? Games Health J. 2015;4(1):31–7.

50. Neri SG, Cardoso JR, Cruz L, Lima RM, De Oliveira RJ, Iversen MD, Carregaro RL. Do virtual reality games improve mobility skills and balance measurements in community-dwelling older adults? Systematic review and meta-analysis. Clin Rehabil. 2017;31(10):1292–304.

51. Johnson D, Deterding S, Kuhn KA, Staneva A, Stoyanov S, Hides L. Gamification for health and wellbeing: a systematic review of the literature. Internet Interv. 2016;6:89–106.

52. Verschueren S, Buffel C, Vander SG. Developing theory-driven, evidence-based serious games for health: framework based on research community insights. JMIR Serious Games. 2019;7(2):e11565.

53. Parisod H, Aromaa M, Kauhanen L, Kimppa K, Laaksonen C, Leppänen V, Pakarinen A, Smed J, Salanterä S. The advantages and limitations of digital games in children's health promotion. Finn J eHealth eWelfare. 2014;6(4):164–73.

54. Barlet MC, Spohn SD. Includification: a practical guide to game accessibility. Charles Town, WV: The Ablegamers Foundation; 2012.

55. Rauti S, Parisod H, Aromaa M, Salanterä S, Hyrynsalmi S, Lahtiranta J, Smed J, Leppänen V. A proxy-based security solution for web-based online eHealth services. In: International Conference on Well-Being in the Information Society. Cham: Springer; 2014. p. 168–76.

56. Graafland M, Dankbaar M, Mert A, Lagro J, De Wit-Zuurendonk L, Schuit S, Schaafstal A, Schijven M. How to systematically assess serious games applied to health care. JMIR Serious Games. 2014;2(2):e11.

57. Robinson TN, Banda JA, Hale L, Lu AS, Fleming-Milici F, Calvert SL, Wartella E. Screen media exposure and obesity in children and adolescents. Pediatrics. 2017;140(Suppl 2):S97–S101.
58. Straker L, Abbott R, Collins R, Campbell A. Evidence-based guidelines for wise use of electronic games by children. Ergonomics. 2014;57(4):471–89.
59. Ferguson CJ. Do angry birds make for angry children? A meta-analysis of video game influences on children's and adolescents' aggression, mental health, prosocial behavior, and academic performance. Perspect Psychol Sci. 2015;10(5):646–66.
60. Hart GM, Johnson B, Stamm B, Angers N, Robinson A, Lally T, Fagley WH. Effects of video games on adolescents and adults. CyberPsychol Behav. 2009;12(1):63–5.
61. Kuss DJ, Griffiths MD. Online gaming addiction in children and adolescents: a review of empirical research. J Behav Addict. 2012;1:3.
62. Peng W. Gaming. In: Thompson TL, editor. Encyclopedia of health communication. Philadelphia, PA: Sage Publications; 2014.
63. Barnum CM. Usability testing essentials: ready, set … test! Amsterdam: Elsevier; 2010.
64. International Organization for Standardization. ISO 9241-11: Ergonomic requirements for office work with visual display terminals (VDTs): Part 11: Guidance on usability. Geneva: ISO; 1998.
65. Kaufman D, Roberts WD, Merrill J, Lai TY, Bakken S. Applying an evaluation framework for health information system design, development, and implementation. Nurs Res. 2006;55(2):S37–42.
66. Yen PY, Bakken S. Review of health information technology usability study methodologies. J Am Med Inform Assoc. 2012;19(3):413–22.
67. ISO. I. 13407: Human-centred design processes for interactive systems. Geneva: ISO; 1999.
68. Bowen DJ, Kreuter M, Spring B, Cofta-Woerpel L, Linnan L, Weiner D, Bakken S, Kaplan CP, Squiers L, Fabrizio C, Fernandez M. How we design feasibility studies. Am J Prev Med. 2009;36(5):452–7.
69. McIntyre A. Participatory action research. Philadelphia, PA: Sage Publications; 2007.
70. Thompson D, Bhatt R, Lazarus M, Cullen K, Baranowski J, Baranowski T. A serious video game to increase fruit and vegetable consumption among elementary aged youth (Squire's Quest! II): rationale, design, and methods. JMIR Res Protoc. 2012;1(2):e19.
71. Thompson D, Baranowski T, Buday R, Baranowski J, Thompson V, Jago R, Griffith MJ. Serious video games for health: how behavioral science guided the development of a serious video game. Simul Gaming. 2010;41(4):587–606.
72. Novak J. Game development essentials: an introduction. Boston, MA: Cengage Learning; 2011.
73. Craig P, Dieppe P, Macintyre S, Michie S, Nazareth I, Petticrew M. Developing and evaluating complex interventions: the new Medical Research Council guidance. BMJ. 2008;337:a1655.

Implementation of Digital Health Interventions in Practice

Lisa McCann and Roma Maguire

Introduction

Digital Health increasingly pervades healthcare delivery worldwide as it offers a plethora of opportunities to provide low cost and high scalability solutions to support healthcare delivery [1]. The WHO define Digital Health as the use of digital and mobile technologies to support health system needs [2]. Technologies supporting Digital Health interventions include mobile phones, wearables, remote monitoring systems, sensors, Virtual Reality, Augmented Reality and data analytics (including predictive risk modelling, Artificial Intelligence and Big Data) and more. Digital Health offers a smorgasbord of technologies which can be utilised individually or in combination with one another to provide innovative patient, carer and clinical models of care appropriate for all aspects of healthcare systems, particularly focused on more efficient health and care delivery.

Digital technologies are 'driving the evolution of healthcare' ([3]: e1). The technological revolution, referred by the World Economic Forum in 2016 as the fourth Industrial Revolution [4], means technologies penetrate many aspect of society and the way we live—from internet banking to online retail—but until recently, technological penetration of the health and care sector was somewhat lagging behind. However, recent developments in which science and technology have converged, many of which were expedited during the global COVID-19 pandemic in 2020, have resulted in the development of innovative digital health devices, products, services and interventions.

L. McCann (✉) · R. Maguire
Digital Health & Care, Digital Health & Wellness Group, Department of Computer and Information Sciences, University of Strathclyde, Glasgow, Scotland
e-mail: lisa.mccann@strath.ac.uk; roma.maguire@strath.ac.uk

© Springer Nature Switzerland AG 2020

A. Charalambous (ed.), *Developing and Utilizing Digital Technology in Healthcare for Assessment and Monitoring*,
https://doi.org/10.1007/978-3-030-60697-8_10

127

Indeed, digital health has emerged as a disruptive and transformational approach to delivering healthcare services as information and communication technologies have real potential to address health needs at scale [5]. Digital Health affords many an ideal opportunity to empower patients, citizens and informal caregivers by providing them with the tools to make meaningful contributions to their healthcare experiences, including accessibility to quality, safe and sustainable healthcare services [6]. Traditional models of healthcare delivery tend to have the clinician as the key stakeholder in patients care, whereas modern and digitally supported approaches to healthcare delivery instead prioritise a collaborative and partnership approach between patients and their clinicians [7]. Meskó and colleagues [7] identified at least nine key differences between traditional and modern healthcare as a consequence of the transformative effects of digital health on healthcare models and delivery, ranging from those less radical (collaborative, rather than hierarchical models of care) to those more so (including point of care testing being the patient, rather than in a clinic or lab).

This chapter will draw on this evolving landscape of digital health service provision and focus on the implementation of digital health technologies in practice by introducing some example frameworks to guide these activities and highlighting some successfully implemented digital health technologies in practice.

Therefore, by the end of this chapter, readers will:

- Develop an understanding of Digital Health
- Understand co-design and participant engagement in the design and development of digital solutions and interventions
- Develop an understanding of theoretical frameworks used to develop, design, implement and evaluate digital health interventions

Understanding Context and Target Users

To design and develop effective digital health interventions, detailed consideration needs to be paid to the users of these technologies and interventions. Human behaviour is complex, and as such, designing digital health interventions must be cognisant of factors such as users' motivations, abilities, resources and social and physical environments [1]. Indeed, a key factor in determining the successful implementation of digital health interventions is ensuring that they have been developed in response to real world need and that key stakeholders such as citizens, patients, carers and health and care professionals have been equal and active partners in the co-design of the product [8]. The central assumption underpinning user co-design is that people are 'experts' in their own experiences and are therefore valuable contributors in defining the function, flow and content of a digital health intervention. Co-design uses the combined creativity of a group as opposed to an individuals and is claimed to result in the development of digital health interventions that are 'more persuasive, feasible, and relevant to users' [9].

For many digital health interventions, user co-design only occurs in the initial stages of product development when in fact it should be a central feature that is active throughout its lifespan. Co-design should be viewed as a constant, iterative and ongoing process, where feedback from key users is used to adapt and modify interventions to respond to the often rapidly changing health and care landscape [10]. As such, regular feedback on the perceptions of key users should be commonplace and importantly used to ensure that the intervention is continually meeting the needs of the population/s that it is designed to serve [11].

Additionally, user co-design should be considered when adapting existing digital health interventions for use in different populations and geographical locations. Different health conditions often give rise to unique needs, and variations in the organisation and delivery of health and care are commonplace from region to region and country to country. For many digital interventions, it is not simply a 'plug and play'—understanding and adaptation of the intervention to the context in which it is being used is extremely important [12, 13, 36]. Understanding perspectives of the population and distinctions of the geographical context are fundamental to ensure successful implementation and ultimately scaling up of the product beyond its original scope and locality.

Theoretical Frameworks to Aid and Guide Implementation

Within the context of implementation science, theories, models and frameworks are now increasingly prioritised as mechanisms to support successful implementation practices [14]. Implementation theories, models and frameworks tend to be cross-discipline and may originate from psychological, sociological, organisational or technological backgrounds; there are now so many different positions on which to draw, and knowing which is the right one to choose can actually prove challenging in itself [14].

Indeed, Nilsen's [14] narrative review of theories, models and frameworks used in the implementation science field identified three **overarching aims** of implementation sciences and five categories of *theoretical approaches* used in implementation science.

- **To translate research into practice**: *Process models*
- **To understand and/or explain influences on implementation outcomes**: *Determinant frameworks, Classic theories and Implementation theories*
- **To evaluate implementation**: *Evaluation frameworks*

The range of models, theories and frameworks identified and categorised by Nilsen [14] is too vast to summarise within this chapter, but readers are advised to review the Nilsen [14] paper in full for further knowledge acquisition in this area.

For the purposes of this chapter to introduce implementation frameworks, four implementation frameworks used in the context of developing and/or implementing (digital) health interventions are briefly summarised.

These are:

- PARiHS
- NASSS
- NPT and NOMAD
- IDEAS

Promoting Action on Research Implementation in Health Services (PARiHS)

Promoting Action on Research Implementation in Health Services (PARiHS) is an implementation model that proposes successful research implementation as a function of the interplay/relationships amongst the nature of '*evidence*', the '*context*' in which the proposed change is to be implemented and the type of 'facilitation', i.e. the mechanism by which change is facilitated to ensure a successful change processes [15–17]. From the perspective of Conklin and Stolee [18], the PARiHS framework is mobilised through three key mediators, defined as:

1. Evidence: Methodologically sound and robust research evidence, clinical experience that has been made explicit and confirmed through consensus amongst practitioners, inclusion of patients in the decision-making process and/or consideration of patient experience.
2. Context: The setting or environment in which evidence is to be used, and is characterised by culture, leadership and evaluation.
3. Facilitation: Conceptualised as the process involved in promoting or enabling research uptake. Facilitators are instrumental in influencing the implementation process, taking into consideration the strength of the evidence and the receptiveness of the respective context [19].

Further Information

Within the PARiHS framework, successful implementation is represented by the following:

$SI = f(E, C, F)$

where:

SI = Successful Implementation

f = function

E = Evidence

C = Context

F = Facilitation

So, **S**uccessful **I**mplementation is a function of the nature and type of **E**vidence, the qualities of the **C**ontext in which evidence is being introduced and the way the process is **F**acilitated [17].

Non-adoption Abandonment Scale-up, Spread, Sustainability Framework (NASSS)

The Non-Adoption Abandonment Scale-up, Spread, Sustainability (NASSS) Framework [20] was developed in response to challenges with achieving routine, scaled and sustainable adoption of potentially impactful technological innovations in the context of health and social care provision. Cognisant of the complexities associated with mainstream implementation of technological innovations, Greenhalgh and colleagues [20] sought to develop an evidence-based, theoretically informed and pragmatic framework that could be used to explore and understand the successes of health and social care programmes that were driven by technological interventions and innovations.

Thus, the emergence of the NASSS framework, developed from a robust systematic review and extensive interrogation of exemplar technology, supported case study programmes. Seven key domains (defined as simple, complicated or complex) relevant to the complexities of adoption of technologies were characterised following the authors' thorough immersion in the various data sources. The seven different domains of the NASSS Framework are:

1. The condition
2. The technology
3. The value proposition
4. The adopter system (staff, patient and lay caregiver[s])
5. The health or care organisation(s) (including attention to the work of implementation and adaptation)
6. The wider (institutional and societal) context
7. Interactions and adaptations over time

Greenhalgh and colleagues argue that NASSS is important as it provides a clear framework in which to explain not only the positive adoption of technologies but also understandings for non-adoption and abandonment [20, 21]. For those concerned or involved in the scaling up of implementable digital health innovations, NASSS provides a framework to understand issues surrounding scalability of digital interventions. If progression from singular and local deployments of digital health innovations to routine use across a locality area (thereby demonstrating scalability) is a practice-orientated concern, then NASSS may prove a useful implementation framework for readers to adopt in their own practices. So too it may prove useful in scenarios where existing successful digital health interventions are to be utilised in different settings to those in which the successes have already been demonstrated (thereby demonstrating spread) and can illustrate maintained use over time (thereby demonstrating sustainability) [20, 22].

Further Information

To aid the application of the NASSS framework, the NASSS-CAT (Complexity Assessment Tool) was developed to provide a range of practical tools to inform understandings, developing, monitoring and research of technology-driven projects and programmes of work in health or social care settings [23]. The NASSS-CAT tools are freely available for download direct from Professor Trish Greenhalgh's website (https://www.phc.ox.ac.uk/team/trish-green-halgh) under the NASSS-CAT Tool sub-heading.

These free-to-access tools include:

- Short and long versions of a questionnaire to guide and reflect on implementation planning,
- An instrument to monitor complexity in technology implementation over time,
- An interview guide and prompts which can be utilised in evaluation interviews with users throughout the implementation processes.

The NASSS-CAT resources provide a robust, evidence-based set of tools which can be used to help practitioners, researchers and technologists plan, conduct and evaluate a technology-supported project or programme of work which focuses on technologically driven service delivery and models of care in both health and social care settings.

Using such tools may generate what is often referred to as 'messy' data, but Greenhalgh et al. [23] argue that this is a strength rather than criticism of the NASSS-CAT tools as these data reflect the realities of the complexities of health and care technology-enabled projects.

Normalisation Process Theory (NPT) and Normalisation Process Theory Measure (NoMAD)

Normalisation Process Theory (NPT) is a sociological toolkit developed to enable researchers to consider issues associated with implementation when designing, developing and evaluating complex (technology-enabled) interventions [24, 25]. NPT was developed to provide a framework to identify factors which promote or prevent routine adoption of complex interventions in everyday practice and is primarily focused on three central issues often associated with the way change and new models of thinking and working are operationalised in healthcare settings, namely [25]:

- **Implementation** (the social organisation of new practices into action)
- **Embedding** (the ways in which new practices do or do not become routinely incorporated into the daily work of individuals and groups)
- **Integration** (the ways in which new practices become reproduced and sustained within an organisation or institution)

NPT, therefore, can be utilised to explain how interventions work, right from their early implementation to their larger scale embedding and normalised use in routine practice. To help explain this, four main constructs are defined within NPT [24, 25] to help explain the actions associated with embedding of practices:

- Coherence (or sense-making): What people do to make sense of a practice.
- Cognitive participation (or engagement): What people do to engage and support a new practice.
- Collective action (work done to enable the intervention to happen): What people do to engage and support a new practice.
- Reflexive monitoring (formal and informal appraisal of the benefits and costs of the intervention): What people do to reflect on and evaluate enacting a new practice in context.

Within the context of health technology innovation and embedding of new practices, NPT has been used as the orienting framework in technology-driven programmes of work across a variety of settings and within the context of various technologies including clinical decision support systems in primary care settings [26], digital self-management programmes for type 2 diabetes [27, 28], and general health and wellness [29].

Further Information
To read more about NPT and to access an online version of the NPT toolkit for use in clinical practice when designing, developing, implementing and evaluating a possible digital health intervention, visit the NPT Interactive Toolkit online. This toolkit can be used to help users consider the different stages of implementation and integration in healthcare contexts and is accessible here:
    http://www.normalizationprocess.org/npt-toolkit/
    In this online resource, the authors have simplified the four NPT constructs into 16 items representing the core values of the theory.
    This is an accessible tool and for each of the 16 items, the following exist:

- A statement that defines the NPT variable
- A sliding bar to input information about the variable
- An explanation which gives more detail about what the statement means

    Consider using the interactive NPT Tool to think through implementation and integration problems in healthcare, to think critically about an implementation problem and at any stage of the implementation process, including from initial thoughts about an idea to understanding the outcomes of implementing a particular digital health intervention.

With NPT's focus on implementation and normalisation of complex interventions, the NPT framework has since been extended to include the development of a specific instrument to measure participants' experiences to implement change and explore the factors associated with the likelihood of normalisation and routine adoption of new practices [30, 31]. The NPT-driven NoMAD instrument (Normalisation MeAsure Development) provides a way to more formally assess, monitor and measure the range of factors that can impact normalisation of new practices by focusing specifically on implementation participation [30]. A potential advantage of the NoMAD tool is the flexibility it affords in terms of how it can be used (i.e. the tool can be adapted) but such adaptations should always only be done in ways that 'make sense' for its targeted participants and relative to the targeted setting of choice. Mishuris and colleagues [26], for example, utilised the NPT toolkit to assess barriers and facilitators associated with the implementation of two new clinical decision support systems in primary care settings. Focused on four implementation domains, the NPT toolkit allowed the authors to longitudinally explore what the implementation barriers were of the new clinical decision support system, thereby identifying areas where further activities were required to further support successful adoption of the new digitally orientated practices.

Further Information

To read more about NoMAD, visit http://www.normalizationprocess.org/nomad-study/how-to-use-nomad/

NoMAD is a 23-item survey focused on assessing implementation processes and can be used in a wide range of purposes and across different settings. It offers flexibility and possibilities for adaptations to explore ways in which digital technology interventions impact on participants' workload, work processes and workflow and likelihood of these new practices becoming normalised into a routine part of their work and associated activities. NoMAD can be used longitudinally over time to explore changes and can be used to improve implementation processes by identifying areas where further work is required to best facilitate progress [30].

In addition, for further information about NoMAD and a range of other international implementation projects, visit the ImpleMentAll website https://www.implementall.eu/17-nomad.html.

ImpleMentAll is a large-scale, cross-European collaborative project funded by the EU Horizon H2020 programme and is focused on faster and more effective implementation of eHealth interventions. Read more about this programme of work here: https://www.implementall.eu/.

IDEAS (Integrate, Design, Assess, and Share)

The IDEAS framework was designed in response to challenges experienced by Digital Health innovators and academics in terms of developing effective digital health interventions that actively facilitate sustainable health behaviour changes

[32]. Designed to encompass multiple core approaches leading to effective digital health interventions, the IDEAS framework provides a step-by-step process to guide the development and evaluation of these digital tools and solutions [32]. Similar to many other implementation frameworks, IDEAS was developed by a multi-disciplinary team from academic, innovation and technological backgrounds, thereby adding to its robust and systematic development processes. Defined by ten phases grouped across four overarching stages, the framework lends itself as an accessible framework for those concerned with the development and evaluation of digital health behaviour change interventions [32].

Within the IDEAS framework [32], the ten key phases and four stages of effective digital health intervention development and implementation are considered to be:

Integrate (insights from users and theory)	1. Empathise 2. Specify 3. Ground
Design (iteratively and rapidly with user feedback)	4. Ideate 5. Prototype 6. Gather 7. Build
Assess (rigorously)	8. Pilot 9. Evaluate
Share	10. Share

The IDEAS Framework is advocated as an appropriate framework to support the conceptualisation, design and evaluation of behavioural change digital health interventions that meet the needs of unique groups of users (e.g. paediatric populations [33]) and specific health behaviours (e.g. increased vegetable consumption [34]).

Further Information
Mummah et al. [34] have developed a step-by-step checklist of the ten IDEAS phases to guide adoption of the framework in digital health intervention development and evaluation. A copy of this checklist is available within the Mummah et al. [34] paper to download and use within the context of your own digital health intervention development and evaluation activities.

Digital Health Interventions Implemented in Practice

A common criticism of many promising digital health interventions is that they do not make it past the pilot stages and suffer from 'pilotitis'. Several contributory factors have been identified including lack of resource, inadequate evaluation and not enough attention being paid to implementation in the early stages of intervention development. It is gradually being recognised that the way in which a digital health intervention is implemented is just as important as the features and functions that sit within it [27]. However, despite this recognition, only a minority of published papers on digital health interventions report on their implementation and lessons learned during this process, limiting understanding and the evidence base to date.

Examples of papers focusing on the implementation of digital health interventions include one published by Furlong and colleagues [35] who reported on their 'lessons learned' during the implementation of the mobile phone-based Advanced Symptom Management System, used to remotely monitor and manage the toxicities of chemotherapy [36] across five countries in Europe. In their paper, the research team discuss pragmatic activities that supported the successful implementation of the ASyMS intervention across multiple countries. These activities included a scoping review of clinical guidelines to ensure that the system was evidence based and aligned to local, national and European practice and the formation of a clinical forum (with representatives from each clinical site) that met regularly to transparently and openly discuss any problems experienced and find solutions to challenges faced. They also highlighted the importance of high-quality and rigorous linguistic translation and validation of various components of ASyMS (patient handset, clinician portal) into the respective native languages to ensure that users could easily understand and use the system within their various countries. The team also described how they developed a practical checklist which was used to confirm the 'readiness' of each clinical site to successfully use ASyMS within clinical care. Components of the checklist included: testing the reliability of data and Wi-Fi networks in each location; assessment of staff competencies following training to ensure that they could satisfactorily carry out simple tasks such as registering and training patients to use the system and dealing with alerts; checking data transfer between the study server and peripheral devices such as the patient handset and clinician portal and ensuring that each site has clearly defined roles and responsibilities prior to implementation.

Ross and colleagues [27] reported on the implementation of the HeLP-Diabetes (Healthy Living for People with Type 2 Diabetes) digital self-management platform which was introduced into 34 GP practices within routine NHS care. Using the NPT as a framework [37], they describe how they developed and adopted a systematic approach to implementation planning and delivery which was informed by systematic reviews of the literature to firstly understand the barriers and facilitators to digital health intervention implementation and secondly to identify evidence-based solutions to address them. Their plan for implementation consisted of activities such as the involvement of key stakeholders including health professionals and clinical commissioning groups; execution starting from small-scale testing before moving onto larger populations and the need for ongoing evaluation and agile adaptation of plans as the process of implementation progressed.

Similar insights into implementation were reported by Dugstad et al. [38] as part of a longitudinal 4 year implementation of a digital night surveillance intervention used in residential care for people with dementia. Findings from qualitative interviews with key stakeholders highlighted several barriers and facilitators to implementation. Relative to the pre-implementation phase the authors reported barriers including: lack of inclusion of 'key actors' in the early phases of the project; an underappreciation of the involvement of the intervention at a wider organisational level; shortage of assessment of risks associated with technology use and patient safety; lack of clarity of roles and responsibilities and an underappreciation of financial and staff resource required to run and deliver the intervention. Interestingly, whilst co-creation was a central part of their early implementation plan, they reported that users, particularly those within the residential care home setting, were not familiar with the principles of user co-design, expecting a fully developed and tailored technology to be provided at short notice. In their paper, the authors cited this as a barrier particularly in the early stages that required time and resource to overcome and for partners to contribute to the development of the intervention in a meaningful way. Additional barriers encountered included digital skills and competencies, instability of the technology and challenges with the delivery and installation of the systems within the residential care home settings, particularly in the early stages of the project. In terms of facilitators to implementation a number of effective strategies were identified including regular workshops organised by the project team which acted as a vehicle for effective communication between the respective stakeholders and a place to share knowledge and find solutions to common problems faced. Establishing a team of project champions was viewed as being an effective mechanism to overcome the barriers to implementation experienced. Throughout, user co-creation was viewed by the authors as being the 'most prominent' facilitator enabling incremental change over time resulting in the delivery of a safer night monitoring service.

Some of the larger organisational factors influencing digital health implementation identified in the Dugstad study [38] were also observed in the *dallas* (Delivering Assisted Living at Scale) programme—a large-scale national technology programme in the UK that aimed to deliver a broad range of digital services to the public to promote health and well-being [39]. Informed by NPT and one of the largest digital health programmes conducted to date, five key challenges were experienced during the early phases of *dallas* implementation. These challenges included establishing and maintaining large partnerships between multiple stakeholders and organisations from several sectors; continually changing external environments; the challenge of paying sufficient homage to user co-design and at the same time achieving change at scale and pace; branding and marketing issues in consumer healthcare settings and challenges in inter-operability of systems and information governance in the presence of commercial propriety models. Based on these learnings, three key areas for future large-scale implementation of digital health interventions were advocated including longer durations of time for the full benefits large-scale programmes of digital health innovations to be realised and assessment of digital readiness of local economies and settings before commencing any digital health innovation at scale. Furthermore, recommendations also highlighted the need for more attention to be directed to information governance and inter-operability which acts as substantial barriers to delivering innovative digital health technologies at scale.

A subsequent paper by Lennon et al. [40] also based on the *dallas* programme further identified three levels of issues influencing readiness for digital health at scale at macro (market readiness, infrastructure readiness, national policy), meso (organisational) and micro (professional/public) levels. One of the main aims of *dallas* at a macro level was to stimulate the consumer digital health market and this resulted in several tensions being experienced. For example, whilst inter-operability of digital health interventions with NHS systems posed technical difficulties for some companies, several commercial partners viewed such challenges as being a threat to their business models—questioning for example whether they should dedicate company resource to ensuring inter-operability with the NHS or promoting their own individual successful digital health interventions abroad. For some vendors, use of their digital health solutions by people with multimorbidity and frailty was viewed as being too risky with product liability being at the forefront of their concerns—particularly for those products that sat out with the health and care sector. The complexity of accessing the digital health marketplace in the UK was also cited as a barrier particularly for international companies with the landscape described as being hard to navigate. Adding to macro level challenges were observations of national policies, e.g. sharing of health data and IT infrastructures and communications technologies, not being up to speed to support the adoption of digital health at pace and scale.

At a meso level, two main challenges emerged including 'industry' and 'local health service organisational' readiness. In terms of industry readiness, for those companies that sold directly to consumers, there was a reticence to invest in the health and care sector—which could have been due to the lack of a coherent market and relative immaturity of the digital health sector at that time. Industry readiness was also impacted on the conflict between collaboration and competition—with some companies not wanting to share insights and IP. Health service readiness and IT infrastructures also posed a challenge particularly in relation to firewalls, legacy systems and strict privacy rules—which hindered rapid deployment across organisations at scale. The constant changing health and care environment, frequent changing responsibility of digital health services amongst health and care organisations and resource constraints also made change at an organisational level problematic.

In terms of micro level readiness, the workload of health professionals and professional confidence in using digital health technologies and concerns regarding issues such as privacy impeded traction as pace. These issues were further impacted by technical constraints such as access to the internet and firewalls, which further fuelled negative perceptions of the use of digital technologies within their professional roles. Some professionals had concerns about blurring and replacement of their roles by technology acted as a barrier to successful adoption and implementation of technologies. In terms of public readiness, many citizens lacked digital skills or access to devices to use the intended solutions—further providing barriers to the use of digital health technologies at scale.

The findings from *dallas* and other studies reporting on the implementation of digital health solutions highlight the complexity of implementation and its importance in progressing the digital health agenda. For digital health interventions focused on patient and organisational outcomes to be fully realised, it is important for key stakeholders within the field of digital health to focus on implementation at inception and report on lessons learned—the good and the bad—to inform this important agenda moving forward.

Barriers and Facilitators to Digital Health Implementation

Although there is increasing evidence of successful and positive small-scale and localised implementation of digital health interventions, there remain some challenges with the speed at which these same interventions are accepted and adopted within routine practice and thus become implemented at scale. Indeed, as previously noted, in their efforts to understand some of the barriers and facilitators to digital health interventions implemented at scale in the UK-wide *dallas* digital health programme implemented between 2012 and 2015, Lennon et al. [41] conducted a longitudinal evaluation of participant experiences. Findings from this longitudinal evaluation indicated the central theme of readiness defined the scale at which the evaluated digital health interventions were successfully implemented and routinely adopted at scale. Within this orienting concept of readiness, three levels of readiness were identified from this large-scale evaluation [41]:

- Macro: market, infrastructure, policy
- Meso: organisational
- Micro: professional or public

Across this hierarchy of readiness, Lennon et al. [41] identified a range of contributory barriers and facilitators to digital health implementation and these concur with experiences of the efforts of other researchers to reach such heralded echelons of wide-scale implementation and adoption.

As outlined in the previous section 'Digital Health Interventions Implemented in Practice', a number of barriers and facilitators to implementation may pervade implementation efforts. Such barriers and facilitators can be summarised as follows:

Barriers to digital health implementation
- Limited or no understanding of the particular context in which the digital health intervention is being deployed and implemented
- Lack of readiness for change and readiness for technology adoption
- Lack of appropriate infrastructure (both in terms of actual IT and personnel)
- Lack of resource (both budgetary and personnel)
- Lack of clarity surrounding information governance
- Lack of engagement with target end users throughout the digital intervention design, development, deployment and evaluation lifecycle

Facilitators to digital health implementation
- Collaborative, partnership approaches to developing and implementing digital health technologies
- Providing adequate and ongoing training for all users of the digital health intervention and technology, including staff and patients
- Adopting an implementation framework to guide the design, development and implementation practices in the clinical setting
- Evaluation of both or either of (a) the actual digital health intervention and/or (b) the implementation process (as per the NPT framework)

- Identify and action Key Champions or Digital Health Navigators within the Clinical Site to support training of clinicians and patients, support and advocate for changes in care processes resulting from implementation of the digital health technologies
- Public, patient and health professional willingness to adopt new technologies and new approaches to care delivery and management

Conclusion

In this chapter, we have outlined the increasingly important role of digital health technologies in healthcare provision and highlighted the importance of working in partnership with end users in the design, development and implementation of these interventions. The role and scope of technological interventions in healthcare has evolved considerably in recent years, largely in response to traditional and reactive models of healthcare being unsustainable. Instead, demands on healthcare services, the increasing pervasiveness of technology in other sectors of society and the drive towards personalised healthcare have accelerated the potential for digital health interventions to be realised and impactful on people's healthcare experiences, both as recipients and providers of care. To ensure the sustainability of these changes in service models, however, careful consideration of the implementation and adoption landscape in which these service developments will sit is vital. Thus, this chapter has introduced possible frameworks, processes, strategies and reflections from practice that can influence the successful scale and reach of long-term digital health intervention use in health and care contexts.

Regardless of the scale of change associated with the implementation of digital health interventions, the value of sharing implementation experiences (such as reflections on the experiences of deployment, including successes and failures) cannot be underestimated as such conversations are vital to move seamlessly from reactive, top down models of care to ones which are defined by collaborative partnership between patients and clinicians and strive to deliver personalised care experiences as much as possible.

References

1. Wang Y, Fadhil A, Lange JP, Reiterer H. Integrating taxonomies into theory-based digital health interventions for behavior change: a holistic framework. JMIR Res Protoc. 2019;8(1):e8055.
2. WHO. Classification of digital health interventions v1.0: a shared language to describe the uses of digital technology for health. Geneva: WHO; 2018. https://www.who.int/reproductivehealth/publications/mhealth/classification-digital-health-interventions/en/.
3. The Lancet Digital H. A digital (r)evolution: introducing *The Lancet Digital Health*. Lancet Digit Health. 2019;1(1):e1.
4. Forum WE. https://www.weforum.org/agenda/2016/01/the-fourth-industrial-revolution-what-it-means-and-how-to-respond/.

5. WHO. Draft global strategy on digital health 2020–2024. Geneva: WHO; 2020.
6. Powell J, Newhouse N, Boylan A-M, Williams V. Digital health citizens and the future of the NHS. Digit Health. 2016;2:2055207616672033.
7. Meskó B, Drobni Z, Bényei É, Gergely B, Győrffy Z. Digital health is a cultural transformation of traditional healthcare. mHealth. 2017;3:38.
8. Trischler J, Dietrich T, Rundle-Thiele S. Co-design: from expert- to user-driven ideas in public service design. Public Manag Rev. 2019;21(11):1595–619.
9. Yardley L, Morrison L, Bradbury K, Muller I. The person-based approach to intervention development: application to digital health-related behavior change interventions. J Med Internet Res. 2015;17(1):e30.
10. Council DH. Design principles for digital health.
11. Steen M. Co-design as a process of joint inquiry and imagination. Des Issues. 2013;29(2):16–28.
12. Ospina-Pinillos L, Davenport T, Mendoza Diaz A, Navarro-Mancilla A, Scott EM, Hickie IB Using Participatory Design Methodologies to Co-Design and Culturally Adapt the Spanish Version of the Mental Health eClinic: Qualitative Study J Med Internet Res. 2019;21(8):e14127. https://www.jmir.org/2019/8/e14127, https://doi.org/10.2196/14127.
13. Craig P, Petticrew M. Developing and evaluating complex interventions: reflections on the 2008 MRC guidance. Int J Nurs Stud. 2013;50:585.
14. Nilsen P. Making sense of implementation theories, models and frameworks. Implement Sci. 2015;10:53.
15. Kitson A, Harvey G. Methods to succeed in effective knowledge translation in clinical practice. J Nurs Scholarsh. 2016;48:294–302.
16. Rycroft-Malone J. The PARIHS framework—a framework for guiding the implementation of evidence-based practice. J Nurs Care Qual. 2004;19:297–304.
17. Kitson AL, Rycroft-Malone J, Harvey G, McCormack B, Seers K, Titchen A. Evaluating the successful implementation of evidence into practice using the PARiHS framework: theoretical and practical challenges. Implement Sci. 2008;3:1. http://www.implementationscience.com/content/pdf/1748-5908-3-1.pdf.
18. Conklin J, Stolee P. A model for evaluating knowledge exchange in a network context. Can J Nurs Res. 2008;40:116–24.
19. Hutchinson AM, Wilkinson JE, Kent B, Harrison MB. Using the Promoting Action on Research Implementation in Health Services framework to guide research use in the practice setting. Worldviews on Evidence-based Nursing. 2012;9(1):59–61. https://doi.org/10.1111/j.1741-6787.2011.00238.x.
20. Greenhalgh T, Wherton J, Papoutsi C, Lynch J, Hughes G, A'Court C, et al. Beyond adoption: a new framework for theorizing and evaluating nonadoption, abandonment, and challenges to the scale-up, spread, and sustainability of health and care technologies. J Med Internet Res. 2017;19(11):e367.
21. Greenhalgh T, Wherton J, Papoutsi C, Lynch J, Hughes G, A'Court C, et al. Analysing the role of complexity in explaining the fortunes of technology programmes: empirical application of the NASSS framework. BMC Med. 2018;16(1):66.
22. Greenhalgh T, Abimbola S. The NASSS framework - a synthesis of multiple theories of technology implementation. Stud Health Technol Inform. 2019;263:193–204.
23. Greenhalgh T, Maylor H, Shaw S, Wherton J, Papoutsi C, Betton V, et al. The NASSS-CAT tools for understanding, guiding, monitoring, and researching technology implementation projects in health and social care: protocol for an evaluation study in real-world settings. JMIR Res Protoc. 2020;9(5):e16861.
24. Murray E, Treweek S, Pope C, MacFarlane A, Ballini L, Dowrick C, et al. Normalisation process theory: a framework for developing, evaluating and implementing complex interventions. BMC Med. 2010;8:63.
25. May CR, Mair F, Finch T, MacFarlane A, Dowrick C, Treweek S, et al. Development of a theory of implementation and integration: normalization process theory. Implement Sci. 2009;4:29.

26. Mishuris RG, Palmisano J, McCullagh L, Hess R, Feldstein DA, Smith PD, et al. Using normalisation process theory to understand workflow implications of decision support implementation across diverse primary care settings. BMJ Health Care Inform. 2019;26(1):e100088.

27. Ross J, Stevenson F, Dack C, Pal K, May C, Michie S, et al. Developing an implementation strategy for a digital health intervention: an example in routine healthcare. BMC Health Serv Res. 2018;18(1):794.

28. Dack C, Ross J, Stevenson F, Pal K, Gubert E, Michie S, et al. A digital self-management intervention for adults with type 2 diabetes: combining theory, data and participatory design to develop HeLP-diabetes. Internet Interv. 2019;17:100241.

29. McGee-Lennon M, Bouamrane M-M, Grieve E, O'Donnell CA, O'Connor S, Agbakoba R, et al. A flexible toolkit for evaluating person-centred digital health and wellness at scale. Cham: Springer; 2017.

30. Rapley T, Girling M, Mair FS, Murray E, Treweek S, McColl E, et al. Improving the normalization of complex interventions: part 1 - development of the NoMAD instrument for assessing implementation work based on normalization process theory (NPT). BMC Med Res Methodol. 2018;18(1):133.

31. Finch TL, Girling M, May CR, Mair FS, Murray E, Treweek S, et al. Improving the normalization of complex interventions: part 2 - validation of the NoMAD instrument for assessing implementation work based on normalization process theory (NPT). BMC Med Res Methodol. 2018;18(1):135.

32. Mummah SA, Robinson TN, King AC, Gardner CD, Sutton S. IDEAS (Integrate, Design, Assess, and Share): a framework and toolkit of strategies for the development of more effective digital interventions to change health behavior. J Med Internet Res. 2016;18(12):e317.

33. Fedele DA, McConville A, Moon J, Thomas JG. Topical review: design considerations when creating pediatric mobile health interventions: applying the IDEAS framework. J Pediatr Psychol. 2018;44(3):343–8.

34. Mummah SA, King AC, Gardner CD, Sutton S. Iterative development of Vegethon: a theory-based mobile app intervention to increase vegetable consumption. Int J Behav Nutr Phys Act. 2016;13:90.

35. Furlong E, Darley A, Fox P, Buick A, Kotronoulas G, Miller M, et al. Adaptation and implementation of a mobile phone–based remote symptom monitoring system for people with cancer in Europe. JMIR Cancer. 2019;5(1):e10813.

36. Maguire R, Fox PA, McCann L, Miaskowski C, Kotronoulas G, Miller M, et al. The eSMART study protocol: a randomised controlled trial to evaluate electronic symptom management using the advanced symptom management system (ASyMS) remote technology for patients with cancer. BMJ Open. 2017;7(5):e015016.

37. May C, Fitch T. Implementing, embedding and integrating practices: an outline of normalisation process theory. Sociology. 2009;43:535–44.

38. Dugstad J, Eide T, Nilsen ER, Eide H. Towards successful digital transformation through co-creation: a longitudinal study of a four-year implementation of digital monitoring technology in residential care for persons with dementia. BMC Health Serv Res. 2019;19(1):366.

39. Devlin AM, McGee-Lennon M, O'Donnell CA, Bouamrane M-M, Agbakoba R, O'Connor S, et al. Delivering digital health and well-being at scale: lessons learned during the implementation of the dallas program in the United Kingdom. J Am Med Inform Assoc. 2016;23(1):48–59.

40. Lennon MR, Bouamrane M-M, Devlin AM, O'Connor S, O'Donnell C, Chetty U, et al. Readiness for delivering digital health at scale: lessons from a longitudinal qualitative evaluation of a national digital health innovation program in the United Kingdom. J Med Internet Res. 2017;19(2):e42.

41. Lennon MR, Bouamrane MM, Devlin AM, O'Connor S, O'Donnell C, Chetty U, et al. Readiness for delivering digital health at scale: lessons from a longitudinal qualitative evaluation of a national digital health innovation program in the United Kingdom. J Med Internet Res. 2017;19(2):e42.

Challenges and Future Directions: From Panacea to Realisation

Andreas Charalambous

Introduction: Setting the Scene

The use of technology in providing and delivering healthcare is pervasive worldwide primarily aiming to monitor, prevent, screen, diagnose, and treat health-related issues on the healthcare and public health level [1]. There are a growing number of technological solutions being introduced in healthcare such as telehealth, electronic health records (HER), Artificial Intelligence (AI), Blockchain technology, digital imaging, robotic surgery, Virtual and Augmented Reality (VR and AR), to name a few. The spread of technology has not only been recorded in terms of the types of solutions implemented but also in terms of the settings where these have been introduced. Over the years the introduction of such technological solutions has not been confined to the hospital context but it has been extended to include remote rural areas, the community, and the patients' home, whilst the use of such technologies has been made possible by means of remote access.

There is an emerging body of evidence in the literature demonstrating that the introduction and utilisation of technological solutions is not without limitations and challenges. There is however an oxymoron, that arises at this point. The factors that are acknowledged as limitations to the technological solutions, can also become their greatest strengths once these are properly addressed. At this point it should be clarified that not all of the presented challenges and limitations are pertinent to every available technological solution or in every clinical context. However, most of the presented limitations and challenges are somewhat common. It is evident in the literature that these can vary significantly with some posing greater threats compared

A. Charalambous (✉)
Nursing Department, Cyprus University of Technology, Limassol, Cyprus

University of Turku, Turku, Finland
e-mail: andreas.charalambous@cut.ac.cy

© Springer Nature Switzerland AG 2020
A. Charalambous (ed.), *Developing and Utilizing Digital Technology in Healthcare for Assessment and Monitoring*,
https://doi.org/10.1007/978-3-030-60697-8_11

to others. In terms of the introduction of technology, preceding research demonstrated that there are challenges in terms of limited access to capital; inadequate broadband and Internet infrastructure; health IT workforce shortages; organisational and cultural challenges, including workflow issues; and security concerns [2, 3]. Ensuring the safety of technological solutions in health and its use in the clinical setting has also emerged as a key challenge [4]. The scientific community is attempting to better understand the complex interactions between people, processes, environment, and technologies as they endeavour to safely develop, implement, and maintain the new digital infrastructure [5]. Another challenge that needs to be considered in the context of utilising technology in healthcare is the level that such interventions correspond to the patient's (i.e. user's) needs promoting a person-centred approach [6]. Technological solutions can raise a number of ethical problems stemming from the inherent risks of devices that can collect and store data on clouds, the sensitivity of these health-related data, and their impact on the delivery of healthcare. A primary challenge of these technological solutions (i.e. especially those that retrieve sensitive patient data) is to ensure that devices and protocols for sharing the data that they create are technologically robust and scientifically reliable, while also remaining ethically responsible, trustworthy, and respectful of user rights and interests [7].

System-Level Challenges from an Organisational Perspective

The discussion on the system-level challenges with regard to the development and implementation of technological solutions within the context of the organisation is undertaken in light of the 'dynamic health system' framework proposed by van Olmen et al. [8]. Based on this framework, health systems are considered as social dynamic systems which are composed of many actors and organisations that interact with each other. The framework incorporates ten elements and their dynamic interactions: (1) goals and outcomes; (2) values and principles; (3) service delivery; (4) the population; (5) the context; (6) leadership and governance; and (7–10) the organisation of resources (i.e. finances, human resources, infrastructure and supplies, knowledge and information).

Essential to the interactions are the elements of communication, coordination, and regulation [9]. These non-linear interactions primarily are manifested between three components, namely service delivery, leadership and governance, and resources within the shifting population needs and contexts and align with a set of values and principles. Technological solutions and knowledge-based tools such as computerised medical records, telecare, or patient decision aids fall within 'knowledge and information systems'. [10].

With reference to the system-level challenges in service delivery although several issues have been identified in the literature, access has been the prevailing issue [11]. Access in this context can have a wider meaning and be related to issues such as limited funds to develop the appropriate infrastructure and technological solutions, limited availability of technological solutions to a limited number of users whilst restrained funding can lead to poor person-centred design and development [10]. The allocation of appropriate funds to put in place the infrastructure to support for example telemedicine (e.g. video consultation), e-prescribing, and the electronic exchange of key clinical information with other providers is of paramount importance to creating the appropriate circumstances to expand the digital culture of a healthcare organisation.

The transformation of healthcare systems in the digital era has seen an unprecedented availability of medical information online or through telemedicine whilst monitoring of the patient and the delivery of therapeutic interventions can be done remotely (e.g. telemedicine, Virtual Reality). Patients now have access to their own medical records and may communicate with their providers using email or online portals rather than needing to visit a facility. Therefore in a changing healthcare context, access can no longer refer only to physical access; for many purposes, it can mean virtual access through telecommunications. Although inadequate broadband and Internet infrastructure can jeopardise to a degree the (e.g. quality, availability) access to these technological solutions, statistics show that with over 4.55 billion people worldwide using a mobile phone in 2014, mHealth apps and interventions will not only continue to empower users but their impact will eventually become universal. Though not everyone will own a smartphone, everyone or very close to everyone will have access to Internet-based information. Access may be through low-cost personally owned devices, community-based Internet kiosks, or some other mechanism [12].

The traditional models of care that rely on health workers, who are taught to diagnose and treat patients and communicate with them about their illness and wellness, are being challenged by a transforming care context where healthcare professionals are required to provide care in new settings, in many times without their physical presence and within a highly digital environment (e.g. with an impact on workflow, nature and scope of their tasks, skills, and responsibilities). Current healthcare systems are already faced up with healthcare personnel shortages, which according to the Global *Strategy on Human Resources for Health: Workforce 2030* [13] can mount up to 9.9 million physicians, nurses, and midwives globally by 2030. The increased demand for effective health workers to master the technical knowledge and skills required to provide high-quality care within such highly digital environments is expected to exacerbate these shortages. For example, studies show that the rapid technological changes which impacted on older nurses' practice competence were identified as a factor for leaving work [14, 15]. Studies also showed that the lack of competency in modern medical technologies can lead to a growing lack of trust in them by the patients [16]. This stresses the need to increase not only older nurses' but all healthcare workforces' access to continuing professional development activities and provide a supportive working environment that cultivates the integration of technological solutions in daily practice.

Several reports by the WHO have acknowledged the importance of leadership and governance as a critical lever for health system development [17–19]. Leadership and governance refer to a government's various roles in health policy ranging from policy implementation to community engagement, including coordination with private and public organisations whose activities impact population. Similar governance issues rested with the development of high-level comprehensive health policies that appropriately regulate the use of technological solutions and digital innovations. The need for health policies that manage expectations and comprehensively and accountably regulate the dissemination, use, and reimbursement of such technological solutions and innovations becomes salient [10]. Beyond the macro level issues of policy-making served primarily by the government, at a micro level, healthcare organisations also play a vital role in the successful introduction and implementation of technological solutions and digital innovations.

Challenges from the User's Perspective

Safety

The issue of safety has been a major concern for many of the emerging technologies and for a number of reasons including the development of safe technology, safe use of technology, and use of technology to improve safety. Safety in this context is a complex issue that is entrenched not only in situations where technology is implemented but as early as its development and field testing. Therefore the process and sustainability of improving the overall safety of the evolving healthcare systems represent a monumental sociotechnical challenge.

The aim of any health technological solution that is designed and developed must be in such a way that it supports the user's needs, preferences as well as goals and workflows. The degree of acceptance (i.e. by the user) as well as the adherence in relation to the utilisation of such technological solutions will be influenced by the level that the technological solution corresponds to the user's specific needs and expectations. From the healthcare organisations' perspective what is essential to be considered is the need to configure appropriately any technological solutions that have been adopted from commercially available products, and ensure that their implementation in various clinical contexts is safe [20]. Promoting and maintaining the safety aspect of these adopted technological solutions needs to take into consideration several issues. For example, their operation corresponds to the design intentions and in cases of on-demand requests (e.g. requests throughout the day and night) by the users, these should be available when and where it is needed.

Another issue to be considered within the safety context is the correct and complete utilisation of the technological solution by all healthcare providers as they care for their patients. It is important for the solutions to be implemented by all those involved in the care as inconsistent use might pose threats to the patient's safety. In those cases that the correct and appropriate use of the technology does not support (or poorly supports) users' needs, preferences as well as goals or existing workflows, then both the software and the workflows need to be reviewed and potentially modified to facilitate safe and effective care [5].

The electronic health records (EHR) provide the possibility to retrieve data that can be useful in monitoring and optimising such technological solutions. Therefore this aspect is stressing for the need for more collaboration of healthcare organisations and electronic health records vendors to enable the technology to help them identify, measure, and improve the quality and safety of the care provided [21].

The utilisation of technological solution in healthcare also presents numerous opportunities for improving and transforming healthcare which includes improving patient safety by reducing for example human errors. In a systematic review, Alotaibi et al. [22] summarised the current available scientific evidence on the impact of different health information technologies on improving patient safety outcomes. The authors concluded that there is extensive evidence that implementing an electronic health record (EHR) reduces medical errors and improves patient's safety. On the same topic, a meta-analyses on the impact of electronic health records on healthcare quality and patient safety demonstrated that institutions utilising these records showed improved guideline adherence, lower medication errors, and lower rates of adverse drug reactions [23].

Other technological systems that have favourable results in improving patient safety include computerised physician order entry (CPOE) and clinical decision support (CDS). Computerised physician order entry relies on the use of electronic or computer support to enter physician orders including medication orders using a computer or mobile device platform. These systems are usually complemented by a clinical decision support system (CDS), which acts as an error prevention tool through guiding the prescriber on the preferred drug doses, route, and frequency of administration [24]. Meta-analyses on the topic showed the effectiveness of these systems in reducing medication errors and adverse drug events in hospitals [25].

Privacy

Personal privacy is not directly related only to control of data but it also includes physical and social aspects that although distinct concepts they are interrelated. In the literature there are many interpretations of what constitutes personal privacy; however for the purpose of this chapter we emphasised on those that are more pertinent to the context of technological solutions. From the physical perspective, privacy can be determined by the physical accessibility of a person to others, defined by physical borders [26] or as the right to be left alone or not monitored by a third party [27]. From the social perspective, personal privacy concerns control over social interaction through geographical distance, group membership, and location [28].

Data produced by technological solutions (e.g. H-IoT, EHR) create opportunities to advance the diagnosis, treatment, and prevention of diseases, and to foster healthy habits and practices among individual users and broader populations [7]. These data may also further the understanding of the contributing factors to disease and the efficiency and effectiveness of treatments and health organisations. Realising these opportunities requires responsible and permissive design of digital data collection tools, analysis, and sharing protocols. During the phase of actual utilisation of such technological solutions and also thereafter, challenges of ethical concern arise with regard to storage, access, sharing, and ownership of data. There are many issues to be considered in the process of maintaining and safeguarding (sensitive) data protection. With regard to informational privacy, this should ensure that personally identifiable data are hidden from any unauthorised parties. Health data in their majority are considered as highly sensitive (i.e. from an ethical and legal perspective), and therefore informational privacy should hold a central place for the design and implementation of technological solutions, insofar as it contributes to gain control over the spread of information about the user's health status and history [29]. Moreover, data have to be stored in such a way that no unauthorised access through hacking or other fraud is facilitated that allows for discrimination and stigmatisation, when confidential information is falling into the wrong hands [30]. What also needs to be considered is the importance of using the retrieved data only for the purpose intended in the first place when consent was granted by the patient/user. Although the initial risks and benefits (i.e. in the context of the retrieved data) of adopting specific technological solutions can reasonably be presented to potential users, the future utility and invasiveness of the data cannot be known (or fully known) at the point of adoption which challenges the current traditional models of informed consent. Therefore these traditional models of informed consent are not directly applicable to many of the data retrieved by many of the emerging technological solutions. Additionally, emerging technological devices can also generate 'invisible data' for which the user is unaware of the scope or granularity of parameters being measured [31] is an aspect which gives cause for concern.

An aspect that can pose as a threat to the social aspects of personal privacy is the possibility that the utilisation of technological solutions (e.g. telemedicine) can contribute to the social isolation of users. In cases where the daily monitoring of health status is controlled remotely there might be a limitation of the face-to-face meetings from the healthcare professionals only in emergency situations or limit to infrequent follow-up visits. Although some technological solutions (e.g. assistive homecare robots) have been proposed as solutions to social isolation, the criticism remains whether such solutions sufficiently and adequately replace interactions between users and human carers [32].

In the era of technological evolution the issue of privacy has become a complex and challenging aspect to appropriately address in healthcare. Although privacy might seem to be threatened by many aspects introduced by digital solutions there are ways to address it effectively in a way to protect the rights of the user. Therefore, the development of user agreements that fairly represent the uncertain value of data generated by users, and the potential for aggregation and linkage by third parties for both research and commercial purposes present as a rather 'solomonic' solution to the threat posed to privacy [7].

Dignity

Dignity is a complex concept subject to a range of different interpretations; however the definition proposed by the Social Care Institute for Excellence provides the appropriate context in relation to the scope of this chapter: '*Dignity is at the heart of personalisation. Dignity means treating people who need care as individuals and enabling them to maintain the maximum possible level of independence, choice and control over their own lives. It means that professionals should support people with the respect they would want for themselves or a member of their family*' [33]. Human dignity, a term often used in health (care) debate, also constitutes a legal concept that, to some extent, can be understood as the crucial minimum requirement for ensuring the protection of every individuals' self-respect in society [34].

Bearing in mind the ethical principle of dignity and as the definitions above stresses also autonomy, the design and implementation of technological solutions needs to take into consideration these principles. In those cases where the dignity of the patient cannot be preserved or can only be preserved to an extent, the implementation of such technologies should be avoided until further actions can be taken to protect the patient/user.

In the context of utilising telemedicine in hospital settings for example, the conveyance of potentially bad news to the patient (or the family and significant others) should be made in keeping the dignity of the patient and promoting his or her autonomy (e.g. power of decision over the means to receive the information). Therefore in this context, distant technologies (through using screens) should be refrained from when delivering news which put the patient in a vulnerable situation [30]. Transferring the control over to the patient for choosing his or her preferred channel of communication, in this specific scenario, there might be a preference towards a more personal and face-to-face communication. This action pathway safeguards not only the dignity of the patient but it also empowers his or her autonomy—in terms of patients' choice of the communication channel—that can contribute to tailoring the delivery of healthcare to patients' needs (i.e. patient centredness).

From a different perspective, patients who do not want to be institutionalised or want to spend the remaining time of their lives (e.g. in palliative care and end-of-life situations) can stay at home longer and be better supported in their home environment by means of technological solutions. Their quality of life and dignity can therefore be increased through the use of such technologies [30]. There is an emerging body of literature that emphasises on the argument that technological solutions (i.e. healthcare robots) can be viewed as a means to help individuals achieve a threshold level of all of the capabilities necessary to maintaining their dignity [34–36]. This perspective acknowledges the fact that although dignity is inherent in every individual, some do not have the mental or physical capabilities to maintain it independently. This can be demonstrated for example in the context of degenerative diseases (e.g. Alzheimer's) where persons can have a severe mental impairment that prevents them from satisfying to the full their basic needs. In this context, protecting human dignity must be a positive obligation for the state, to ensure that these people in question get the help they need to achieve the minimum level of self-respect and self-worth, guaranteed by human dignity. Therefore in these cases, technological solutions can be utilised to support the person in fulfilling his or her basic needs, promoting this way ones sense of self-respect and self-worth.

Threat to Person-Centredness

The positive impact of technological solutions is evident in the context of hospitals in effective patient monitoring over time and improved communication with patients; and in positive experiences among professionals and patients. Despite its positive effect on these aspects of healthcare, there is scepticism about the impact on person-centredness and person-centred care. Furthermore, for the development of technological solutions, user-focused techniques (e.g. usability testing) are still used infrequently—if at all. Finally, while person-centred care, by definition, argues for tailoring solutions for the specific needs of each person, digital solutions in traditional care are designed around a set of standard patients' pathways seen from a medical perspective [37].

There are various challenges to developing and implementing technological solutions in healthcare that have a 'humanising focus'. The first challenge is to clearly articulate what a humanising focus entails and maintain its manifestation as a primary focus for practice in this digital age [38, 39]. Across the different technological solutions, various challenges have also been identified from a technical perspective. The inability of the technological solutions to adjust to the personalised needs of the patients, the inability to integrate patient-driven information (e.g. in non-formative text), limited responsiveness to patient's changing health status, data fragmentation, and poor interaction with the patient are only some of the issues that have been identified as technical limitations to implement person-centred care [40].

As discussed in Chapter "Personalizing the Technological Experience", recognising the way in which humans interact with technologies, not abstract properties of technology, is essential to achieving changed practices and systems of care, enabled by technology, to drive better health outcomes. The necessity to focus on the 'human factors' in relation to technological solutions has driven key developments in the field spanning intervention development, implementation, and the quest for patient-centred care. What becomes apparent is that the key to successfully integrating the human factors in the design, development, and utilisation of technological solutions is consistency in their utilisation [6]. Adopting a person-centred approach (e.g. a true co-design approach) to developing and implementing technological solutions can also address some of the barriers to improved health outcomes. Therefore a technological solution that has been developed according to the patient's needs (or is responsive to patient's needs) can increase user engagement (and adherence) with mobile health interventions. Furthermore, the patient can have a more positive attitude towards sharing personal information via such solutions (i.e. to be utilised within a care pathway) especially when those information increase their empowerment via an increased control over the decision-making process. Finally, these personalised technological solutions create the conditions where the patient is more likely to integrate such solutions at their home context as a means to avoid hospitalisation and maintain their autonomy (e.g. via better self-management).

Conclusion

Digital health is a field that is emerging and constantly evolving. As a result the challenges in their totality surrounding its design, development, and implementation are impossible to identify and incorporate in any implementation strategy. As new questions and challenges emerge, their incorporation to the design and implementation strategies will need to be made accordingly over time.

These challenges however do not minimise the potential of such technological solutions when applied in practice. The aim should be to create the proper conditions that will make people capable of actually using the opportunities offered to them if they wish. This can be achieved through the provision of accurate and truthful information about the benefits and risks of engaging in the utilisation of technological solutions within healthcare. This empowering strategy (which should also include the family and significant others) provides the appropriate motivation to the users to engage in digital health technology. Any empowering strategy to be considered complete in this context should not only support the provision of information but also to support the technical skills of the users. Therefore for this to be achieved, open communication, technical training, and education should be provided. Another issue that needs to be considered in this process is that any participation by the user should be voluntary. Moreover their voluntary participation should not be undermined by any sort of incentive, be it of financial nature or prioritising those that use digital health technologies when they seek medical care in non-digital, conventional healthcare settings.

Technological solutions can have a transformation impact on health systems in various ways including broadening health coverage and spreading health information and literacy, reducing healthcare costs, and promoting efficiency to report a few. However, we need to acknowledge that technological solutions in health also catalyse challenges with regard to digital illiteracy, resulting in significant inequities in access and informed consent, which need to be addressed. Therefore, it is crucial for all stakeholders, especially digital health providers, to ensure that the digital health interventions are designed and utilised in an ethical and fair way, thus fostering equity in access and fair equality of opportunity for all population groups and taking into account the needs of disadvantaged groups.

Technology should not be viewed as a panacea within the healthcare context but rather as a tool that can facilitate the provision of care and one that presents itself with strengths and limitations. Designing, developing, and implementing person-centred technological solutions can be facilitated by comprehensively understanding the interactions between technology and its users. These processes provide a clear agenda for digital health research in the quest to identify and address barriers to desired health outcomes. It also provides a warrant for the value of this research domain at a time when the ubiquity of information technology might otherwise make digital technologies 'just another' delivery mechanism for intervention or systems change.

References

1. Currie WL, Seddon JJ. A cross-national analysis of eHealth in the European Union: some policy and research directions. Inf Manag. 2014;51:783–97.
2. Maust D. Implementation of an electronic medical record in a health system. J Nurses Staff Dev. 2012;28(1):E11–5.
3. Gabriel MH, Jones EB, Samy L, King J. Progress and challenges: implementation and use of health information technology among critical-access hospitals. Health Aff. 2014;33(7):1262–70.
4. Kim MO, Coiera E, Magrabi F. Problems with health information technology and their effects on care delivery and patient outcomes: a systematic review. J Am Med Inform Assoc. 2017;24(2):246–50.
5. Sittig DF, Wright A, Coiera E, Magrabi F, Ratwani R, Bates DW, Singh H. Current challenges in health information technology–related patient safety. Health Informatics J. 2020;26:181. https://doi.org/10.1177/1460458218814893.
6. Huckvale K, Wang CJ, Majeed A, et al. Digital health at fifteen: more human (more needed). BMC Med. 2019;17:62. https://doi.org/10.1186/s12916-019-1302-0.
7. Mittelstadt B. Ethics of the health-related internet of things: a narrative review. Ethics Inf Technol. 2017;19:157–75. https://doi.org/10.1007/s10676-017-9426-4.
8. van Olmen J, Criel B, Bhojani U, Marchal B, van Belle S, Chenge MF, Hoerée T, Pirard M, Van Damme W, Kegels G. The health system dynamics framework: the introduction of an analytical model for health system analysis and its application to two case-studies. Health Cult Soc. 2012;2(1)
9. van Olmen J, Criel B, Van Damme W, et al. Analysing health systems to make them stronger. Stud Health Serv Organ Policy. 2010;27:2–98.
10. Lehoux P, Roncarolo F, Silva HP, Boivin A, Denis JL, Hébert R. What health system challenges should responsible innovation in health address? Insights from an international scoping review. Int J Health Policy Manag. 2019;8(2):63–75.
11. Kostkova P. Grand challenges in digital health. Front Public Health. 2015;3:134.
12. Mitchell M, Kan L. Digital technology and the future of health systems. Health Syst Reform. 2019;5(2):113–20.
13. WHO. Global strategy on human resources for health: workforce 2030. https://www.who.int/hrh/resources/globstrathrh-2030/en/.
14. Valencia D, Raingruber B. Registered nurses' views about work and retirement. Clin Nurs Res. 2010;19(3):266–88.
15. Uthaman T, Chua TL, Ang SY. Older nurses: a literature review on challenges, factors in early retirement and workforce retention. Proc Singapore Healthcare. 2016;25(1):50–5.
16. Sheiman IM, Shishkin SV. Russian health care: new challenges and new objectives. Probl Econ Transit. 2010;52(12):4–49.
17. World Health Organization. The World Health Report 2000: health systems: improving performance. Geneva: World Health Organization; 2000.
18. World Health Organization. Everybody's business–strengthening health systems to improve health outcomes: WHO's framework for action. Geneva: World Health Organization; 2007.

19. World Health Organization. The World Health Report 2008: primary health care: now more than ever. Geneva: World Health Organization; 2008.
20. Sittig DF, Singh H. Electronic health records and national patient-safety goals. N Engl J Med. 2012;367(19):1854–60.
21. Singh H, Sittig DF. Measuring and improving patient safety through health information technology: the health IT safety framework. BMJ Qual Saf. 2016;25(4):226–32.
22. Alotaibi YK, Federico F. The impact of health information technology on patient safety. Saudi Med J. 2017;38(12):1173–80. https://doi.org/10.15537/smj.2017.12.20631.
23. Campanella P, Lovato E, Marone C, Fallacara L, Mancuso A, Ricciardi W, et al. The impact of electronic health records on healthcare quality: a systematic review and meta-analysis. Eur J Pub Health. 2016;26:60–4.
24. Agency for Healthcare Quality & Research. Computerized provider order entry. https://psnet.ahrq.gov/primers/primer/6/. Accessed 2020.
25. Nuckols TK, Smith-Spangler C, Morton SC, Asch SM, Patel VM, Anderson LJ, et al. The effectiveness of computerized order entry at reducing preventable adverse drug events and medication errors in hospital settings: a systematic review and meta-analysis. Syst Rev. 2014;3:56.
26. Bowes A, Dawson A, Bell A. Ethical implications of lifestyle monitoring data in ageing research. Inf Commun Soc. 2012;15(1):5–22.
27. Dorsten AM, Sifford SK, Bharucha A, Mecca LP, Wactlar H. Ethical perspectives on emerging assistive technologies: insights from focus groups with stakeholders in long-term care facilities. J Empiric Res Hum Res Ethics. 2009;4:25–36. https://doi.org/10.1525/jer.2009.4.1.25.
28. Bagüés SA, Zeidler A, Valdivielso F, Matias R. Sentry@ Home-Leveraging the smart home for privacy in pervasive computing. Int J Smart Home. 2007;1:129–46.
29. Baldini G, Botterman M, Neisse R, Tallacchini M. Ethical design in the internet of things. Sci Eng Ethics. 2018;24:905. https://doi.org/10.1007/s11948-016-9754-5.
30. Brall C, Schroder-Back P, Maeckelberghe E. Ethical aspects of digital health from a justice point of view. Eur J Pub Health. 2019;29(Suppl 3):18–22.
31. Bietz MJ, Bloss CS, Calvert S, Godino JG, Gregory J, Claffey MP, et al. Opportunities and challenges in the use of personal health data for health research. J Am Med Inform Assoc. 2016;23(e1):e42–8.
32. Wu YH, Fassert C, Rigaud AS. Designing robots for the elderly: appearance issue and beyond. Arch Gerontol Geriatr. 2012;54:121–6.
33. The Social Care Institute for Excellence. http://www.scie.org.uk/publications/guides/guide15/index.asp. Accessed 10 Mar 2020.
34. Zardiashvili L, Fosch-Villaronga E. "Oh, Dignity too?" said the Robot: human dignity as the basis for the governance of robotics. Mind Mach. 2020;30:121. https://doi.org/10.1007/s11023-019-09514-6.
35. Nussbaum MC. Frontiers of justice: disability, nationality, species membership. Cambridge: Harvard University Press; 2009.
36. Sharkey A. Robots and human dignity: a consideration of the effects of robot care on the dignity of older people. Ethics Inf Technol. 2014;16(1):63–75.
37. Islind AS, Lindroth T, Lundin J, Steineck G. Co-designing a digital platform with boundary objects: bringing together heterogeneous users in healthcare. Heal Technol. 2019:1–14.
38. Galvin KT, Todres L. Caring and well-being: a lifeworld approach. London: Routledge; 2012.
39. Health Education England and the Royal College of Nursing. Improving digital literacy. 2017. https://www.rcn.org.uk/professional-development/publications/pub-006129.
40. Burridge L, Foster M, Jones R, Geraghty T, Atresh S. Person-centred care in a digital hospital: observations and perspectives from a specialist rehabilitation setting. Aust Health Rev. 2018;42:529–35.